yoga
JOURNAL

PRESENTS

YOUR GUIDE TO
REIKI

D0067311

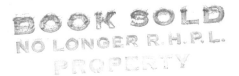

Adam

57 Li

nc.

S.A.

Contains mater   uide to Reiki by
Phylameana   Media, Inc.,
ISBN 10: 1-440   5-2787-6.

ISBN 10: 1-4405-9384-1
ISBN 13: 978-1-4405-9384-0
eISBN 10: 1-4405-9385-X
eISBN 13: 978-1-4405-9385-7

Printed in the United States of America.

10 9 8 7 6 5 4 3 2 1

This book is intended as general information only, and should not be used
to diagnose or treat any health condition. In light of the complex, individual,
and specific nature of health problems, this book is not intended to replace
professional medical advice. The ideas, procedures, and suggestions in this
book are intended to supplement, not replace, the advice of a trained medical
professional. Consult your physician before adopting any of the suggestions in
this book, as well as about any condition that may require diagnosis or medical
attention. The author and publisher disclaim any liability arising directly or
indirectly from the use of this book.

Many of the designations used by manufacturers and sellers to distinguish their
products are claimed as trademarks. Where those designations appear in this
book and F+W Media, Inc. was aware of a trademark claim, the designations
have been printed with initial capital letters.

Cover design by Sylvia McArdle and Frank Rivera.
Cover images © iStockphoto.com/DragonImages/Kontrec/Paul Whittle.
Interior illustrations by Kathy Konkle.

This book is available at quantity discounts for bulk purchases.
For information, please call 1-800-289-0963.

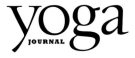

PRESENTS

YOUR GUIDE TO
REIKI

Use This Powerful Healing Energy to
Restore Your Body, Mind, and Spirit

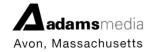

Avon, Massachusetts

CONTENTS

INTRODUCTION

REIKI IS A SIMPLE AND NATURAL system of touch healing that originated in Japan through the discovery of a Zen Buddhist named Mikao Usui. The history and healing techniques used in Reiki are continuously passed down from teacher to student through a unique attunement process. Today, there are a variety of different lineages, all of which stem from this one man's influence.

Although Reiki is a spiritual healing art, it is not associated with any one belief system or doctrine, organized or otherwise. For this reason, Reiki practitioners make up a very diverse community. Reiki can be practiced by anyone who is open to its love energies. All that you need in order to give yourself a Reiki treatment are your hands, your body, and a willingness to touch it. Regardless of the status of your health, whether you are incredibly healthy or troubled by disease or injury, Reiki can offer great benefits. When you are ill, Reiki treatments can help restore you to good health. When you are healthy, Reiki treatments will reinforce your vitality and strengthen your immune system.

Reiki is a holistic healing modality that encourages relaxation and relieves suffering. Its gentle action makes it a perfect instrument to have readily available under all circumstances. As you learn and begin to use Reiki, you will discover that it is easily accessible in any situation because it "turns on" automatically whenever you place your hands either on your body or on another person's body.

Extremely adaptable, Reiki complements other types of health treatments. Pre-op and post-op Reiki treatments will often shorten the care period following surgery because Reiki accelerates the healing process. Also, Reiki treatments can easily be conducted in your home because no special equipment is required. The recipient can relax in a bed or recliner during the session.

This book is meant to present Reiki not only as a healing art, but also as a way of life. Reiki is so simple that Reiki Level I, the first of three levels of training, can be learned in only a few short hours. And yet, after a person takes that first-level Reiki class and becomes attuned to Reiki, he will be changed forever. The changes that may occur will vary from person to person, but these are changes that will ultimately be positive for everyone.

Balance comes to both the giver and receiver of Reiki's ki (life force) energies. In this book, the term "practitioner" is used to represent the person giving a Reiki treatment. The term "recipient" represents the person receiving it. Everyone who has been attuned to any level of Reiki may be called a Reiki practitioner.

Reiki will extend its gentle, yet powerful, healing energies to you. All you have to do is open your heart to it and invite it in.

PART 1

WHAT IS REIKI?

*Be the peace you want to see
in the world.*

Gandhi

In this part, you'll be introduced to the basic concepts of Reiki. You'll find out what it is, where it came from, and how it developed. You'll discover the way it uses ki (life force) energy to help create healing. You'll learn how and where energy enters and leaves the body, and you'll learn about the basic techniques practitioners commonly perform to encourage the flow of this energy where it is needed. You'll also discover what it feels like to perform and receive Reiki treatments and how to measure the Reiki pulse to facilitate flow.

CHAPTER 1

REIKI ENERGY AND SENSATIONS

The energy we give heals our own wounds.

Jaclyn Costello

THE TERM "REIKI" is derived from two Japanese syllables, *rei* and *ki* (pronounced "ray key"), meaning Universal Life Energy. Rei represents the source of this energy and ki represents the energy's movement within and around us. In this chapter, you'll discover more about Reiki energy, how to channel ki, and what experiencing Reiki feels like. You'll also find out the appropriate way to honor Reiki and you'll learn the basic techniques of how to perform Reiki.

Finally, you'll find out more about Reiki sensations, including why you may not experience any at all, why Reiki healers are sometimes said to have "hot hands," and why you may sometimes feel extra hands are helping you.

What Is Reiki?

Usui Reiki Ryoho is an energy healing art that derived from ancient healing practices that intentionally channels ki energies to promote balance and well-being. Ki is the Japanese term that refers to the life force, or living energy, that connects us to everything and sustains our life breath. Ki animates the body and gives life its pulse. Every living thing exists because of ki. Without ki, there is no life. When a person, animal, tree, or any living thing is in poor health, it is an indication that ki is not functioning as well as it could be. A sickly body's energy is blocked in some way, meaning that ki is not able to flow freely. The Reiki practitioner assists the recipient by channeling pure ki energies into the body to help break through blockages and balance his or her life force. It is important to remember that a Reiki practitioner does not "heal" the recipient, but helps the recipient heal himself or herself. A Reiki practitioner is simply a channel for energy that the recipient will use for its highest and best use.

Reiki Is Energy

Reiki is the source of Universal Life Energy, and it is also a term used to describe the healing modality that accesses and transmits that energy. Reiki as a healing instrument operates through the concept that there is an unlimited supply of Universal Life Energy available for us to tap into.

It can be difficult to describe what Reiki is to someone who has not come into contact with it, but it can be helpful to think about how you would describe the wind to someone who has never experienced it. You cannot actually see the wind. You can feel and see only the effects of the wind; you feel its warmth or coolness against your skin when a breeze is gentle, and you see its strength when trees and homes are leveled during hurricanes. Wind upsets your hair, sweeps and scatters leaves about, waves your flags, and so on. It is an external force that you feel outside of your body. In contrast, Reiki could be compared to wind internalized. Reiki's life source fluctuates within your body and can be depleted by physical or emotional stress, but also restored through healing.

Reiki, in its purest form, is basically an uncomplicated system of healing. You do not have to believe in Reiki for it to work. The practitioner cannot claim or take responsibility for healing or nonhealing when Reiki is applied. Reiki works at the level of acceptance of the person who is receiving it. Acceptance is not a matter of faith or belief. Acceptance suggests that there is a willingness to move from a painful experience into a less painful experience.

Reiki As Love Energy

Because of its gentle nature, Reiki is often described as a love energy. Its infinite healing power is limited only by our self-made boundaries. As you open up to Reiki's love energies, you will discover the myriad of benefits it offers, including the following:

- Reiki replenishes vitality of life.
- It treats causes and symptoms of dis-eases.
- It clears away toxic and stagnant energies.
- It serves as a stress reliever and calming agent.
- It boosts the immune system.
- It enhances intuition.
- It does not conflict or interfere with any religious beliefs.
- It complements other healing modalities.
- It is always available, wherever you are.
- It promotes balance in all aspects of your life.
- It offers unconditional love.

How Reiki Enters the Body

Also known as energy vortexes, or wheels of light, chakras are funnel-shaped centers within our bodies that serve as intake and outflow mechanisms to control the flow of ki energies that sustain us. Healers are familiar with seven major and twenty-one minor chakras. Chakras are discussed in more detail in Chapter 17. Reiki enters the body through one or a combination of these centers. Some people believe that Reiki is pulled upward from the earth's grounding energies through the soles of the feet at the earth chakra. Others believe it enters from a celestial source through the top of the head at the crown chakra. Others feel it enters through the tan tien (the energy center located just below the navel, also called the hara or sacral chakra), and some feel it enters through the root chakra (at the base of the spine).

Open and functioning chakras spin clockwise, allowing energy to vitalize our auras and nourish our physical bodies.

How Reiki Flows from the Body

When Reiki is applied to the recipient, healing energies flow out of the practitioner's body through the palms of the hands as they touch the recipient's body. The energy flow varies in speed, depending on various factors such as the extent of the recipient's illness, degree of blockage, and readiness to accept change. The source offers an unlimited supply of Reiki so that we, as facilitators of Reiki, are never depleted.

REIKI REFLECTIONS

Reiki is not a religion. Having a belief system is not necessary for Reiki to work. Reiki does not infringe on your right to believe what you wish and does not require you to change or switch your religious faith. Christians, pagans, agnostics, Hindus, Buddhists, and Jews may freely adopt Reiki as a means to heal and bring harmony into their lives.

How Is Reiki Taught?

Reiki is taught through the process of passing attunements from Master to student. An attunement is best explained as a metaphor. Think of your body as a radio with the power turned on. You have access to energy (or a radio station) all the time. An attunement allows your body to be adjusted like a radio dial so you can hear the station clearly. An attunement clears and opens the channels in your own body so you are now connected to the source of universal ki. Attuned Reiki students are then able to serve as conduits of an unlimited supply of Universal Life Energy that can be transferred to others, assisting them in healing.

Reiki is so powerful that a healer that has had an attunement will notice that life changes start to happen. In order to be a conduit for pure, loving ki energies, you must let go of things that are no longer serving you. Awareness of the possibility of experiencing subtle, and at other times, pronounced, changes in your life as an aftereffect of an attunement will benefit you in the long run.

Before attempting to draw upon this powerful healing reservoir, a person must be able to accommodate it, so that the life force can flow freely. Through the attunement process, a passageway is cleared within the body to serve as an empty vessel for channeling the ki energies.

Keep in mind that in order to become a Reiki practitioner, you must be attuned by a teacher. Some people have proclaimed themselves to be Reiki practitioners without ever having been attuned by a teacher. This is not ethical behavior and dishonors the Reiki rite of passage. However, this is not to say that you cannot tap into the life force and do energy-healing work without being attuned to Reiki. There are other energy-healing modalities that do not involve attunements; however, it is the initiation process involving attunements that makes Reiki different from other energy-healing techniques.

REIKI REFLECTIONS

Much of this book focuses on becoming a Reiki practitioner, how to do self-Reiki, and how to go about giving Reiki treatments to family members or friends. But before you immerse yourself too deeply in the academic aspects of Reiki, and before signing up for a class and becoming attuned to Reiki, schedule a session for yourself with a practitioner and experience it firsthand. Reiki is for everyone, but not everyone is for Reiki. Consider getting at least one or two treatments before agreeing to an attunement.

Reiki Sensations

What does Reiki feel like? As Reiki energies flow between practitioner and recipient during a Reiki session, the two bodies may respond or react with particular sensations. These sensations are nearly always pleasant. You may feel heat, warmth, cold, or sensations of subtleness, steadfastness, or forcefulness. The fact that you can feel Reiki energy flowing, whether you are giving or receiving it, is verification that the energy is being welcomed.

What It Feels Like

Reiki works like a thermostat that regulates the body. Much like a furnace that automatically turns on and off to regulate the temperature, Reiki flows slowly or rapidly—as needed—to dispense balancing energies. Reiki sometimes moves erratically, other times smoothly. These fluctuations of ki energy churning within us can often be felt as pins and needles, hot flashes, goose bumps, throbbing, and so on.

Sensations Felt by Giver and Recipient

During a Reiki treatment, both the Reiki practitioner and the recipient feel sensations. A practitioner's hands will often heat up as a result of the flow coursing through his palms. The recipient frequently feels sleepy and yawns repeatedly as incoming Reiki energies soothe and calm pent-up emotional tension and stress.

REIKI REFLECTIONS

You may experience any of the following sensations during a Reiki session: heat or coolness, pins and needles, tingling, vibrational buzzing, electrical sparks, numbness, throbbing, itchiness, and sleepiness.

Some people are more in tune with their bodies than others and will be able to share fantastic stories about feeling the different sensations that occur while using Reiki. They will talk about experiencing imagery, kinesthesia, and/or inner voices while either giving or receiving Reiki.

For some Reiki practitioners, hand temperature may change as they are giving Reiki treatments. These changes range from burning hot to icy cold. Sometimes, the practitioner's perception and the recipient's perception of the temperature will be different. For instance, as you are giving Reiki, you may feel that you're burning up, but your recipient may feel coolness from your touch. Or, it may be that you are experiencing cold hands, while the recipient may comment on the warmth of your hands.

You May Not Feel Anything

Reiki sensations can be very subtle and may be overlooked, but with continued practice most people will begin to notice even the slightest shifts of energy. A few people will seldom, if ever, feel anything with Reiki beyond the tactile sensation of hands-to-body touch.

Fortunately, Reiki works whether you feel it or not. If you are having difficulty feeling sensations while giving a Reiki treatment, try closing your eyes. Keeping your eyes shut eliminates visual distractions, which will help you focus more on the person and the sensations.

Hot and Cold Hands

It is often taught that after receiving your Reiki Level I attunement, you will develop hot hands. Having hot hands is supposedly a credible sign that the attunement worked and that you are now officially a channel for Reiki. Experiencing hot hands may very well indicate that Reiki has been awakened and you are now a genuine, functioning Reiki conduit. But if you do not experience hot hands, does that indicate nothing has happened and that your attunement was a failure? Not at all. Every person's attunement experience is unique. Being told that you need to experience hot hands or that your experience was somehow deficient because it was different from that of others is greatly misleading.

REIKI REFLECTIONS

Always wash your hands with soap and water before applying Reiki. Avoid fragrant soaps and lotions, especially if the person you are treating may be allergic to the aromatic chemicals used in those products. If your hands are naturally cold, briskly rub your palms together for several seconds to warm them up before beginning treatment.

Extra Healing Hands

This is an experience that is not at all uncommon. Some recipients may feel that additional practitioners are participating in the Reiki session. For instance, one woman reported that during a one-on-one session with the Reiki practitioner, she felt two additional pairs of hands placed upon her body. One explanation of the "extra healing hands" sensation is that healing spirit guides are present. Another explanation is that Reiki goes to the place it is needed most. If a practitioner is placing his or her hands on your crown chakra and you feel like hands are on your stomach, it could be because the Reiki is going directly to your stomach where it is needed. Reiki has an innate intelligence that a practitioner can't control. Your job isn't to control Reiki; it is to be a conduit.

REIKI REFLECTIONS

Maureen J. Kelly, author of Reiki and the Healing Buddha, *says the sensations of the hands that Reiki practitioners experience can be explained by the Chinese philosophy of yin and yang. If the practitioner's hands are hot, it indicates the recipient's body has too much yang energy. If the hands are cold, the body has too much yin energy.*

Vibrating Hands

Water pipes expand and contract to accommodate the water as it flows through them. In this same manner, your body also adjusts to the flow of Reiki being channeled through it. When Reiki is being drawn out of your palms at a faster rate or in larger proportions than you are accustomed to, you may experience your hands vibrating. The vibration occurs as a result of the Reiki gushing through your body so quickly that it gets backed up into your hands. Reiki is trying to get out and go where it needs to go, but the openings in your palms are too narrow to pass it on efficiently. Fortunately, aside from being uncomfortable, the shakiness in your hands is merely signifying that the person receiving Reiki from you is in great need. The recipient is absorbing Reiki as fast as he or she can get it.

Other Sensations

Aside from the vibrational sensation in your hands, you may also experience soreness in your wrists and the joints of your fingers. In treating people with severe illnesses, you may feel a powerful pulling of Reiki energies from your neck, shoulders, and down your arms as well. If you find channeling greater volumes of Reiki painful or uncomfortable when treating someone, periodically remove your hands from the recipient to give your hands a chance to rest. You can alternate—ten minutes hands on, ten minutes hands off, and so on.

CHAPTER 2

THE REIKI PULSE

Look at every path closely and deliberately,
then ask ourselves this crucial question:
Does this path have a heart?
If it does, then the path is good.
If it doesn't, it is of no use.

Carlos Castaneda

THE PULSATING SENSATION OF REIKI can be felt in all parts of your body, but especially in the palms of your hands. This is because the palms are the outlets of Reiki energy. Reiki wants to flow out of your hands and be put to good use. As soon as you place your hands on yourself, or someone else, Reiki automatically turns on. In this chapter, you'll find out more about the Reiki pulse and how to facilitate the flow of Reiki through you to others. You'll also be assured that using Reiki will never deplete you—Reiki is limitless. And you'll learn about the importance of using (and releasing!) empathy in Reiki treatments.

Letting Reiki Flow

After you are attuned to Reiki, you become a walking generator of sorts: Your body will heat up and start spewing out healing energies whenever you are near anyone who is receptive to Reiki. This feeling can overwhelm the newly attuned person, especially if he had not been advised beforehand that this could happen. Your immediate reaction may be to place your hands on the person, but this is not recommended. Never assume that you have the right to approach a person and touch him just because your body's sensations are telling you that he is open to it. Always ask first.

You do not need to lay your hands on the person for Reiki to flow over to him. Simply put a smile on your face and allow Reiki to do all the transference; just being aware that you are a conduit for Reiki is sufficient. The receptive person doesn't need to be aware that anything is happening.

If you are among a crowd of people, such as sitting in a movie theater or shopping at the market, you probably won't be certain to whom the Reiki is actually flowing. Accept your role as a Reiki channel and try not to get caught up in a need-to-know mindset. It is not important to know where the Reiki is going. Simply let it flow. After a while, you won't even pay attention when Reiki is flowing from you because it will become a routine occurrence.

REIKI REFLECTIONS

Healers who are familiar with the healing properties of gemstones will sometimes combine the healing energies of specific crystals in their Reiki sessions with clients. Metals, on the other hand, are conductors of energy and will absorb Reiki, cheating the receiver of the full benefit. Magnetic jewelry also presents a problem, as it polarizes the Reiki energy.

Excess Reiki Energy

There may be times when Reiki will ball up in your hands, creating a circling orb of energy. Imagine having a tennis ball glued to the palm of your hand. No matter how hard you try, you cannot shake it off. Now, imagine that this tennis ball is a living organism that has a pulse.

Experiencing these pulsating balls of energy in your hands can be an odd or even disturbing sensation, but there is nothing to worry about. Reiki isn't flowing anywhere outside of you, because there is no specific place for it to go. However, this may very well be an indication that self-Reiki is needed. Take advantage of this excess of energy in your hands and place your hands on your body. Allowing the Reiki to flow into your body should help reduce or release the ball of energy from your palms.

Anytime you feel an excess of energy building up in your body, you can take advantage of this by infusing inanimate objects with Reiki. Placing Reiki inside objects transforms them into healing instruments. Reiki can be put into any object by holding the object between your hands and allowing Reiki energies to pour into it. Reiki Level II practitioners can also place Reiki symbols, along with their energies, into these objects, making them become even more powerful. Any of the following objects may be filled with Reiki:

- Reiki your bed pillow, filling it with Reiki energies for a restful night's sleep.
- Reiki your bath water—nothing feels more soothing than soaking in a Reiki bath.
- Reiki your lamps and light bulbs—their illuminations will have a Reiki glow!
- Reiki your aromatherapy candles, incense sticks, and flower essences.
- Reiki your shampoo, skin lotions, and toothpaste.
- Reiki your vitamins and prescription medications.
- Reiki your food so that you can absorb its nutrients more efficiently.

- Reiki your computer to reduce the number of system crashes.
- Reiki your telephone to help you be more patient with disruptive callers.

Facilitating the Flow

Reiki flows in the direction of the easiest pathway. When the natural course of a river comes up against a dam, the water pools up in that area until it either breaks through the blockade or reroutes itself by traveling around the obstacle, moving through to the next available open channel.

REIKI REFLECTIONS

Reiki is just like a river. Its energies flow through our bodies, following the most natural path in filling us up. The hand placements used to administer Reiki allow the energy to enter the body through different channels.

There are twelve basic hand placements that are used in giving a full-body Reiki treatment—four placements on the head, four on the front of the body, and four placements on the back of the body. Applying Reiki for five minutes in each of these placements helps to distribute Reiki evenly over the whole body. However, when hands are placed on one area, sometimes the person will experience hot spots elsewhere. For example, you may have your hands placed on the person's throat, yet the person will feel a trickling of energy running down one or both of her legs. Always know that Reiki goes where it needs to go.

Dealing with Blockages

As you move your hands through the various hand placements, you may come to a position on the body that feels blocked. When you no longer feel Reiki flowing from your palms, your first impulse may be to move on to the next hand placement—but hold on. Blocked areas are denser and often need more attention given to them. Sometimes all you need to do is shift your hands an inch or two from that position, either up or down, in order to get Reiki to start flowing again. If this doesn't work, be patient. Keep your hands on the recipient's body where you sense Reiki is being blocked for a full five minutes before moving along.

In Tune with Your Etheric Hand

No pressure is to be applied to the body when giving Reiki. Place your hands gently on the body. However, there may be situations when your hands might feel as if they are actually sinking deeply into the body while giving Reiki. This sinking or magnetic pulling sensation happens when your etheric hand extends itself into the deep tissues.

REIKI REFLECTIONS

During a Reiki treatment, you may sense a waft of fragrance. This can be an indication that a spirit guide, angelic being, or Ascended Master is visiting your session.

Removing your physical hand before your etheric hand has retracted itself to join the physical hand can cause a disruption in the healing session. If your hands feel like they are stuck to the body, it is likely that this kind of deeper etheric healing is occurring. It is advantageous to keep your hands in position for an extended period while this deeper healing work is being done. If it is not feasible for you to keep your hands in position due to time constraints or some other unavoidable reason, be sure to remove your hands slowly without any abrupt movements. Take care to be as gentle as possible.

A Vessel That Never Empties

When you are giving a Reiki treatment to someone, you are giving your time and your intent to assist; you are not giving away any of your own energy. Reiki is in infinite supply. It never runs out. As a Reiki practitioner, you are making yourself available as a vessel through which Reiki can be accessed.

During and after giving a Reiki treatment, you may feel a variety of emotions. These feelings can run the gamut from exhaustion to exhilaration, or something in between. However, these feelings have not occurred because you have been drained of energy. Something else is going on. It is possible that you were in great need of Reiki yourself, and by giving Reiki to another person, you also received Reiki. Reiki will always attend to the practitioner's needs as well as to the recipient's. Reiki always offers a double treatment. If you routinely feel tired after giving Reiki to someone else, this is an indication that you need to focus on self-treatments for a while. After attending to your own needs, you will feel better and more capable of sharing Reiki with others.

If a practitioner is empathic, touching other people may cause her to develop mirrored illnesses. However, having empathic abilities is not a requirement of Reiki, nor does it enhance Reiki's effectiveness. Empaths need to learn that the ability to "take on" or "feel" another person's pain or emotions is best used as a diagnostic tool. Don't hold on to the empathic feelings—they must be released as soon as possible.

People with empathic natures are also known as highly sensitive people, ultrasensitive people, or people with "overexcitabilities." When you find yourself feeling the sensations of someone else's emotions or pains within your own body, take some gentle, deep breaths and ask the person you are treating to take a few deep breaths as well. This should help break up the blocked energy so that you can continue the treatment without continued discomfort.

Perception Techniques

Byosen Reikan Ho and Reiji Ho are two Reiki techniques taught in Japan. These techniques focus the practitioner on perceiving sensations within the body of the person being treated. You can learn how to develop your intuitive abilities and use intent when treating illness and imbalance. The learning process is gradual, as you continue to practice giving Reiki treatments to others.

PART 2

GETTING STARTED IN REIKI

*We are not human beings having a
spiritual experience. We are spiritual beings
having a human experience.*

Pierre Teilhard de Chardin

In this part, you'll take your first steps on your Reiki journey. You'll learn the basics of getting started in this ancient healing art, from finding the appropriate teacher to preparing for your attunement to participating in it. Next, you'll explore Reiki principles and learn how to honor your body temple. Finally, you'll discover how to design the right environment for healing, including pretreatment preparations, setting healing intentions, and creating appropriate expectations.

CHAPTER 3

REIKI ATTUNEMENT PROCESS

In every community, there is work to be done.

In every nation, there are wounds to heal.

In every heart, there is the power to do it.

Marianne Williamson

A REIKI ATTUNEMENT is an expansion process, or, you could say, a knock at the door that opens to a space that already exists. That "space" is a passageway within our bodies through which the Universal Life Energy travels. Receiving a Reiki attunement can be a meaningful or even life-altering experience. The attunement ritual is performed with a Reiki Master/Teacher (someone who is a Reiki Master and has also been taught how to pass attunements on). Choosing the right person to initiate you into the world of Reiki can make all the difference in how you experience your Reiki attunement. In this chapter, you'll discover the steps to take on the first part of your Reiki journey—finding the right Reiki Master/Teacher for you and preparing for your attunement.

Choosing the Appropriate Reiki Master/ Teacher

As you probably remember from past school days, not all teachers are equal. Most people will prefer to study with teachers who have personalities that will not clash with their own, as well as teaching styles that will not be in conflict with their self-images and learning habits. Moreover, people learn best when a teacher displays integrity and a passion for her subject.

REIKI REFLECTIONS

The term "master" implies a person who possesses insightful knowledge and esteemed wisdom. Perhaps this is representative of some Reiki Masters. But most others are bumbling along in life the best way they can, just like everyone else, and don't wish to be regarded as having any special elite status or powers. Respect them, yes, but don't worship them. In Reiki, the title merely means "teacher."

Meeting Prospective Teachers

Interviewing Reiki teachers in order to find the appropriate person to initiate you into the world of Reiki can be almost as frustrating as shopping for the perfect pair of shoes. You may have to try on quite a few before you find the perfect fit. Don't settle for penny loafers when you really have your eye on those crimson leather pumps. Another customer may find the penny loafers quite comfy to wear, but they aren't for you. When choosing your Reiki teacher, take your time and consider your options carefully. The relationship between Reiki teacher and student is not one to take lightly.

The interview does not have to be a lengthy process. A three- to five-minute phone call should provide a sufficient amount of time for you to get either a good or bad feeling about your prospective teacher.

REIKI REFLECTIONS

Don't expect a potential teacher to invest more than about ten minutes of her time in discussions with you before you have committed yourself to signing up for a class. If you wish to speak extensively with a teacher on the telephone, or to meet him or her for an informal interview, ask if remuneration is expected. After all, time is a valued commodity.

Interview Questions

There are certain questions you should first ask yourself and then other questions that are more appropriate for you to ask your potential teacher. Also, be prepared to answer any questions from the teachers you might interview. Keep in mind that the interview can go either way. You might decide to back out first if you sense that a good student-teacher relationship might not be possible, or the Reiki teacher might decline to teach you if she feels that there is not sufficient rapport between the two of you.

Obviously, the Reiki teacher has the final say as to who will or won't become her student. Don't be discouraged if one Reiki teacher refuses you. Consider that it's all for the best, and seek out another possible teacher.

QUESTIONS TO ASK YOURSELF

- Does the teacher's gender matter to me? Do I prefer a male or female teacher?

- Am I willing to travel in order to attend a class? If so, how far away from home am I willing to go?
- How much am I willing to pay for instruction?

QUESTIONS TO ASK POTENTIAL TEACHERS

- What are your credentials? How long have you been working with Reiki?
- How many attunements do you pass to your students? Do you offer booster attunements?
- Are you available for your students after class? To what extent?
- What materials will I need for your classes?
- What topics do you cover in your classes?
- How much classroom time is instructional, and how much is hands-on practice?
- What are your fees?
- What is your Reiki lineage?
- Will I receive a Reiki certificate after completing your class?
- Are you involved in a Reiki group in my area?
- How many students are there in your classes?
- Do you teach all levels of Reiki?
- What Reiki systems do you teach?

Don't be nervous or dwell for long on any second thoughts about the attunements. You'll get through them all just fine. There is so much more to Reiki than the initial empowerment.

Beyond the Interview

Aside from evaluating the responses each potential teacher gave you in answer to your questions, you should also consider how each individual impressed you overall. With which teacher did you feel most comfortable? Who seemed to be the most knowledgeable? Did any of them seem annoyed by your questions?

First impressions are normally good indicators for how the two of you will get along during the class. After all, how helpful can a person be in answering questions you might have during a class if she was brusque or irritable while giving responses to your questions during the initial interview?

Reiki Lineages

"What is your Reiki lineage?" This question, occasionally posed to Reiki practitioners, seems to suggest that some teachers might be better qualified to teach Reiki. But a person's Reiki lineage is merely the progression of Master-student relationship that is traced back, in one way or another, to Hawayo Takata, the teacher most responsible for bringing Reiki to the United States. It is not at all an indicator of how pure or powerful a person's teaching strengths or abilities may be.

Reiki teachers attract students who can learn from them, but Reiki students may also have something to teach their Masters. Don't allow lineage, or lack of lineage, to get in the way of learning Reiki from the most appropriate teacher.

If a particular lineage is important to the student, by all means, the student should procure a teacher who can verify that desired lineage. But, it would be hoped that other factors would also be considered in evaluating a person's knowledge of and familiarity with Reiki.

Preparing for the Attunement

Once you have found your teacher and set up a time for the attunement ceremony, you will need to start preparing your mind and body for the event. Your body should be free of any substances that diminish mental awareness or stimulate the body unnaturally, such as nicotine, caffeine, alcohol, and recreational drugs. Do continue taking any prescribed medications according to your health provider's directions.

A full night's sleep prior to your class is recommended, so get to bed early, or at least avoid any late-night activities like watching television into the wee hours of the morning. Be sure to eat a healthy, nutritious breakfast the morning of your class. Fifteen to twenty minutes of meditation in the morning will also help calm you of any jitters or stomach butterflies.

Reiki Initiation Ritual

The Reiki attunement is much anticipated by Reiki students. Attunements have been and still are somewhat cloaked in secrecy. The Reiki students are requested to keep their eyes shut when the attunements are passed on to them. Naturally, this gives Reiki attunements an air of mystery, implying that the students are not supposed to see what is being done with them. The actual reason that students are asked to keep their eyes closed is to help them achieve a relaxed and meditative state.

The attunement process inspires myriad feelings and emotions. Every newly attuned practitioner's experience of his attunement is unique. It is a personal and intimate experience that some individuals prefer to keep private. Others can barely hold their excitement and will quickly share their Reiki awakening experience with others.

Number of Attunements

Traditional Usui Reiki Master/Teachers give their students four attunements for initiation into Reiki Level I, two attunements for Reiki Level II, and one attunement for Reiki Level III. Attunements for all levels are somewhat similar, but each also has its own slight variation.

In addition to the traditional attunements given by Usui Reiki Master/Teachers, there is a powerful and versatile attunement called the Hui Yin. The Reiki Master/Teacher can use the Hui Yin whenever he feels a student is in need of this special attunement. The Hui Yin is also called the booster attunement.

Reiki and Karma

During or after the attunement ceremony, many Reiki practitioners experience the phenomenon of remembering the use of Reiki in a former life. For some, this memory will surface through their conscious wakeful minds, detailing considerable information. Visually sensitive people might actually witness the scenes being played out through images in their mind's eye. At other times the memory enters through the subconscious mind in nighttime dreams.

Some people feel that those who are drawn to Reiki here on earth were predestined to be healers during times when our planet is suffering unrest and afflictions such as war, poverty, and environmental disturbances.

Twenty-One Days of Purification

After receiving a Reiki attunement, it is completely normal for an individual to go through a detoxification or cleansing period. Your body needs to be cleansed both physically, emotionally, and spiritually so you can be a clear conduit for Reiki. Some people experience physical symptoms such as mild diarrhea, cold or flu symptoms, stomach upset, headache, or mild fatigue. Be sure to drink plenty of water to help with the purification process.

While the physical body is going through its purging process, spiritual and mental detoxification is also taking place. You might notice that old emotions you've bottled up resurface in order for you to deal with and release them. The spiritual body's housecleaning is often expressed by changes in sleep patterns, experiencing vivid dreams, and third-eye openings. The mental body cleanses when the individual's brain reorganizes his thought patterns. It is during this period that self-evaluation takes place and personal healing can begin. After receiving an attunement, you should do a self-treatment every day to help with the purification process and balance your energies. Don't hesitate to get in touch with your teacher if you have questions during the cleansing period.

Coping with Highs and Lows

The highs and lows associated with getting a Reiki attunement can feel like a bit of a roller coaster. Some people feel like they are floating on air, their senses are more keen, that their heart is completely open, and the very next day they are feeling low and in need of some comfort. The best way to adjust to any changes that occur is to be as gentle as possible with yourself. Listen to your body and give it what it asks for. If you are feeling tired, take a midday nap or go to bed early. If you are craving chocolate, indulge yourself and eat a piece of chocolate. Whatever you do, do not deny your body what it craves.

Do your best to cope with any mood swings that you experience. If you feel like crying, allow the tears to flow naturally without trying to stifle the sobs. If you feel like getting in touch with someone you haven't spoken to in a while, do it. Your mind and body are going through a healing at this time as well. Listen to your instincts.

Finding Alone Time

If you need some alone time and your family is crowding you, pack your bag and check yourself in to a hotel room for a couple of days to allow yourself the privacy you need. If the demands of your family don't allow you to escape to a hotel, try some other creative ways to achieve solace, even if only for short periods. Lock yourself inside the bathroom and take a soothing warm soak in the tub. Or you can instruct your family members that whenever you are wearing a particular article of clothing, it signifies that you wish to be left alone. The article you wear should be something that can easily be attached and removed as needed, such as a scarf tied around your neck or a sash around your waist.

The Benefits of Reiki Always Outweigh Temporary Discomfort

After reading about the discomforts and mood swings that can occur during the detoxification period that follows an attunement, you might be wondering why anyone would even want to sign up for a Reiki class. Why put yourself through that pain? Who wants to feel sick? Is there an upside to all this? Do the benefits truly outweigh the possible hardships suffered along the way?

In response to these questions, consider the following. In less than a month's time, your body will become cleared of all those impurities that most likely took you years to accumulate. Having a Reiki attunement is like pushing the speed-dial button on your telephone. It transmits quickly, cutting through any garbling static in the wiring. There is never a wrong number dialed. Reiki knows where to go and how to make the right connection. The connecting party is you.

Each Reaction Is Different

Although the attunement process is the same for everyone, it affects each person in a different way. Some people will glide through the purification period with barely any noticeable changes. Others will go through a more difficult adjustment. It all depends on what condition the student is in prior to the attunement. If you tend to bury your emotions, Reiki will push them to the surface in order to force you to deal with them in the open. If you were suffering from a flu infection that had not yet run its course, Reiki would magnify all your symptoms (chills, fever, and headache) and advance their progression through your body more quickly. This means that you will perhaps suffer from these symptoms more intensely, but the flu will burn itself out in one or two days, rather than linger in your body for a longer period of time.

Similar to Reiki attunements, Reiki treatments can also speed up healing in this same manner. This is why some people will report that they felt worse after receiving a Reiki treatment than they did before the treatment. If there are active imbalances in your body that are menacing to your health, those imbalances can become exaggerated when Reiki is given. Symptoms might quickly heighten to greater degrees than they would have otherwise. But, on the positive side, with Reiki's assistance, those imbalances, magnified or not, will pass entirely out of the body much sooner than expected.

CHAPTER 4

REIKI PRINCIPLES

Your vision will become clear only when you look into your heart. Who looks outside, dreams. Who looks inside, awakens.

Carl Jung

THE REIKI PRINCIPLES, also known as Reiki precepts, are the spiritual ideals of the practice of Reiki. Dr. Mikao Usui, founder of the Usui Reiki System of Healing, added the precepts to his teachings when he realized that Reiki encompassed much more than just the physical aspects of healing. Dr. Usui was a spiritual man. He valued daily prayer and ethical behavior, and he believed that by living these basic principles, a harmonious life would result.

Repeating the Reiki principles daily serves as a basic preparation for treating yourself and others as they should be treated. There are many variations of the Reiki principles in print. Here is one version:

- Just for today, I will not be angry.
- Just for today, I will not worry.
- Just for today, I will give thanks for my many blessings.
- Just for today, I will do my work honestly.
- Just for today, I will be kind to my neighbor and every living thing.

The Reiki principles are spiritual ideals loosely based on the Buddhist teaching to live in the moment with the understanding that it is not what happens to us in life that upsets us but our reactions to life circumstances that can bring about upsets. Living the principles will help you achieve inner peace and harmony.

Cleansing Your Body Temple

Your body serves as the vessel through which Reiki flows to another person. For this reason it is important that your body is clean, well groomed, and nourished when you're giving a treatment.

Shower or bathe your body, brush your teeth, and assure that your breath is freshened before the arrival of the person you intend to treat with Reiki. Use natural or unscented deodorants. Avoid wearing perfumes or washing beforehand with scented soaps, since some people are sensitive to the chemicals in these products.

Epsom salts, sea salts, and baking soda are all body purifiers that can be used effectively in the bathtub. Soaking in a tub filled with warm water with any of these or with a mixture of them for fifteen to twenty minutes will detoxify your body. A detoxification bath will also draw energy from the body and can make you feel drained afterward. Be sure to replenish your energy by drinking eight to twelve ounces of spring water during and/or after the bath.

Take an Aura Bath

Giving yourself an aura bath is great anytime, but it is especially helpful between Reiki sessions. Your aura is like a magnet, picking up vibrational energies that are floating around everywhere you go. It is important to cleanse your aura frequently, freeing it from foreign vibrations and negative energies. Here are three ways to cleanse your aura:

1. Cleanse your hands with cool running water. Then, use your fingers to "comb" through the space surrounding your body, from head to toe. After you're done, cleanse your hands again.

2. Using a single feather or feather whisk made from owl or turkey feathers, make sweeping motions through the space surrounding your body.

3. "Smudge" the area surrounding your body with the smoke from an herbal wand made from white sage, lavender, cedar, and/or sweetgrass. (Avoid doing this if you suffer from any respiratory problems.)

REIKI REFLECTIONS

To smudge your aura: Light the smudging wand using a match or candlelight. Blow the flame out or wave the wand to put out the fire. Allow the smudge stick to smolder, freeing the smoke to circle in the air. Holding the herbal wand in one hand, fan the swirls of smoke with your other hand around your body's aura from your head to your toes.

Soak Up Healing Rays

Sit by a sunny window and soak up some healing rays for a few minutes each morning. The sun is a natural healer and will vitalize your body, fend off depression, and keep your energy balanced. If you live in a region where sunshine is sparse, you can substitute light therapy by sitting under special lamps designed for this purpose.

Dressing Comfortably

The most appropriate clothing to wear, whether you are the practitioner or the recipient, is anything comfortable and loose fitting. Don't wear nylon pantyhose or any type of clothing that clings to the body too tightly. Garments made from natural fabrics

If you are ever asked to remove your clothing to receive a Reiki treatment, immediately consider this an inappropriate request. Refuse any further treatment by the practitioner and head straight for the nearest exit. That Reiki practitioner is not to be trusted.

such as cotton are more breathable than synthetic materials. Nonporous and clingy synthetic fabrics tend to restrict the flow of Reiki. It is not necessary for recipients to remove apparel for Reiki treatments, but they should take off their shoes and belt.

Reiki recipients should wear cosmetics sparingly or not at all. Also, they should avoid using hairspray. Cosmetics and hairspray can be a hindrance, since the hands of the Reiki practitioner will be touching the recipient's face and head.

Nourishing Your Body

Having optimal health is essential for practicing Reiki, and eating well is essential for optimal health. Eating five or six small-portion meals each day is recommended over eating just two or three large meals. Make healthy food choices and avoid all fast foods, snacks loaded with carbs, and junk foods.

Some healers prefer to fast before treating others because the digestion process can interfere with their personal comfort and overall efficiency when doing healing work. If this is the case, be sure to nourish your body after the Reiki session is over. However, you also don't want to experience hunger during the session. A growling tummy can be a distraction, so a small meal beforehand might be called for. Consuming a piece of fruit, a few celery or carrot sticks, a small handful of almonds, or a small glass of fruit juice or bottled water before a session might be enough to stave off hunger pangs.

Certainly keep any of your meals light prior to giving someone a treatment in order to avoid feeling sluggish or having gastrointestinal discomfort. Avoid eating garlic or anything that can cause offensive breath. Do not drink any alcoholic beverages and avoid all caffeinated drinks for at least twenty-four hours prior to giving Reiki.

Drink plenty of purified or natural spring water to keep yourself hydrated.

Be sure both you and the recipient use the bathroom before beginning a Reiki session. A full-body treatment can last from one to two hours, and it is best if neither of you interrupt the session.

Creating a Healing Space

It is meaningful to have a space dedicated to healing. Whether you have a room designated solely for Reiki treatments or only temporarily set up an area as a Reiki space in your home, honor your healing space by keeping it clean and uncluttered. Televisions and telephones have no place in your healing space. Turn the television off and turn off the ringer on your phone.

If you cannot turn off the telephone, inform the Reiki recipient that your answering machine will record any calls if your phone rings and that the Reiki session will not be interrupted. The Reiki session should always be your first priority. Avoid any distractions that might arise suddenly. Taking a phone call or answering the doorbell in the middle of a healing session would give the Reiki recipient the message that he is clearly not your first priority.

Reiki Equipment and Supplies

Keep all your equipment and related supplies close at hand. Here is a list of recommended items to have available:

- Massage table—You can use a bed, couch, or recliner to give a full-body Reiki treatment, but a massage table is the most comfortable choice. There are many portable tables on the market. The standard width is 29 inches. The standard height is adjustable from 22 to 35 inches. You can expect to pay from $300 to $500, depending on the table model that best fits your needs. Or you can find a suitable used table online.

- Face rest—The face rest is an accessory to your massage table. It allows the Reiki recipient to lie face down on his stomach. Without the face rest, the recipient will need to have his neck turned to the right or left, which can cause discomfort after a prolonged period of time. You can also purchase washable covers for the face rest, providing additional comfort and hygiene.

- Chair—You will need a chair or stool to sit on when giving a Reiki treatment. An armless desk chair with wheels or a swivel stool are both good choices so that you can roll back and forth as needed when positioning your hands.

- Bolster—A bolster is used to relieve stress from the lower-back region. Keep the bolster tucked under the Reiki recipient's knees while he is lying on his back. A smaller one can also be tucked under the recipient's ankles when he is lying on his stomach. A makeshift bolster can easily be made by rolling up a large, soft towel.

- Blanket—Keep a blanket or two nearby to cover the person you are treating in case he complains of feeling chilled.

- Pillows—Most recipients prefer to have a pillow cushioning their head, or perhaps a small rolled-up hand towel under the neck, rather than lying with their head flat on the table surface. Pillows can also be used as arm rests for you as you give the treatment. A firm pillow placed on your lap will provide much-needed comfort and prevent cramping or shaking as you stretch your arms across the table and over the recipient's body.

- Other items—Additional supplies to have readily on hand are clean linens, tissues, a wastebasket, and bottled water.

CHAPTER 5

PRETREATMENT PREPARATIONS

*I am open to the guidance of synchronicity, and
do not let expectations hinder my path.*

Dalai Lama

REIKI CAN BE DONE with no preparation whatsoever when treating emergency conditions or providing quick anxiety relief during times of trauma. However, when you're applying a full-body Reiki treatment, you should take a few simple steps in preparation. Preparedness helps you develop focus and intent, and helps the recipient to feel more relaxed and more receptive to healing. In this chapter, you'll learn how to provide the right atmosphere for Reiki, including setting your intentions, creating appropriate expectations, and learning to center and ground yourself.

Setting Healing Intentions

Healing can be strengthened when you have a clear goal to reach. Setting an intention before the treatment begins helps to focus the energy used in healing. So, you should know why the recipient has requested a Reiki healing. That way, both you and the recipient are focused on the same outcome.

Receiving Clarity

Sometimes it is not clear as to why a treatment is needed. When this is the case, you can suggest that the first treatment be focused on the recipient receiving clarity as to what his most significant needs are. Using "receiving clarity" as an intention can be very powerful in getting directly to any illness or imbalance within the body.

The Gassho Ritual

Gassho (pronounced "gash sho") is the act of bringing the hands together in a prayer-like fashion in front of the heart. It is used as an acknowledgment, a prayerful greeting of sorts. In using Gassho, the Reiki practitioner is recognizing the source of the healing energies and is thanking the Creator for the opportunity to serve as a vessel for Reiki to flow through. Gassho is often done for a few brief seconds before the session begins and again at the end of the session. The healing intention that was selected for the session can be stated out loud during the Gassho ritual at the start of the Reiki treatment.

Curbing Your Expectations

Setting an intention is very different from having an expectation. An intention is a focus that empowers healing, allowing it to unfold naturally. An expectation tends to limit healing because holding an expectation is a form of rigid control and involves passing judgment.

Charge up your battery by nourishing your body and doing whatever needs to be done to offer the best help you can. But, aside from that, there is nothing more you can do. Setting up expectations is really only setting up yourself and the recipient for failure.

Being able to put aside your expectations and accepting whatever happens in a healing session is not always easy. As healers, we want to help heal people's dis-eases, but placing an expectation on the "when" or "how" a person will heal is actually a controlling mechanism. We are not in control of anyone's healing journey. We are only facilitators, willing to act as tools.

When you expect someone to get better and they don't, you will feel bad and blame yourself. If you expect nothing and the recipient doesn't get better, you may still feel bad, but you won't blame yourself for the failure of achieving something you expected.

Centering and Grounding

Each one of us has a unique personality, and so we often get caught up in the illusion that we are totally separate beings. But in reality, each of us is only a minuscule part of the whole. We are a part of the universe, not something outside of the universe. Our egos want to keep us isolated from one another when we place overt importance on our differences. However, we can appreciate and celebrate our individual uniqueness without isolating ourselves from the universe.

It is the power of the universal source that sustains us. Yoga and tai chi are two excellent exercise methods that can help align your energies with the universe. Meditation and visualization are other ways that help to center and ground our energies.

REIKI REFLECTIONS

A grounded person is one whose energetic soul body is in sync with the physical body. If you are emotionally charged, either by expression (anger, frustration, sadness) or by experience (bewilderment, distraction, confusion), you are ungrounded, with your soul drifting away to another place. Being accident-prone is an obvious characteristic of being ungrounded.

Guided-meditation CDs and videos can help you become centered and grounded. Look for taped meditations that are meant for chakra alignment or for grounding yourself. Following are a couple of scripted meditations that you can try.

Earth-Grounding Meditation

You are barefoot, sitting on a stone bench alongside a grassy hillside. Focus on your feet. They are touching the ground beneath you. Imagine roots shooting out from the soles of your feet and your toes. Imagine the roots spreading wider and deeper into the soil. These roots enable you to draw into your body the positive energies of the Mother Earth.

Your feet have now sunk into the moist dirt. Wiggle your toes in your comfortable earthy slippers. Notice your ankles being tickled by the tall grasses blowing in a gentle wind. Feel the blood pumping through the veins in your legs.

Feel your buttocks planted firmly on the cool stone bench. Move your hips slightly from side to side, allowing your body to adjust to the natural curvature of the stone. You are now a part of this stone. You are feeling very relaxed.

Relax your breathing. The deeper you breathe, the more relaxed you feel. Continue to take slow, deep breaths. Deep . . . deep . . . deeper. Listen to the constant pulse of your heartbeat. Let the sound of the steady beat of your heart drop to your solar plexus. Belly in. Belly out. Belly in. Belly out.

Release any tension in your back. Allow your torso to slump slightly. Every movement you make releases more and more tension from your body. Move your shoulders slightly forward. Allow your head to wobble gently from side to side. Tip your head to the right. Now tip it to the left. Drop your chin to your chest. Allow your head to bob up and down slowly. Allow your head to wobble naturally, with no jerky motions.

Lift your head. Close your eyes. Focus on your eyelids. Notice the flutter of your lashes against the soft tissue under your eyes. Keeping your eyes shut, allow yourself to notice the movements of your eyeballs. Are they still? Are they moving? Don't force them to do anything; just let them be.

Take your hands and allow your fingers to walk across your scalp and through your hair. Imagine that this tingling sensation is awakening your brain and stimulating your thought processes. Comb your hair with your fingers. Don't worry about messing up your hairstyle. You are now clearing away any debris from your aura that is obstructing your crown chakra. By doing this you are clearing a pathway for you to feed from the universe's unlimited healing energies. With your feet planted deeply into the earth, open your crown to receive the white light pouring down through your crown chakra and into your whole being. . . . You are now aligned with the Creator and ready to begin.

REIKI REFLECTIONS

You can record personal podcast-guided meditations using computer software or with a voice-recording application compatible with your Blackberry, Android, or iPhone. As you record your voice, speak slowly and enunciate.

Ocean-Grounding Visualization

Imagine that you are lying inside a glass-bottomed boat that is floating over the deep blue ocean waters. You are lying on your belly, looking down toward the ocean floor. There are many colorful fish swimming in the water beneath you. You are safe in the boat, yet you feel as if you are very much a part of the marine life—the coral reefs, seaweed, fish, and sea turtles. You can feel the boat rocking gently to the rhythmic motion of the ocean waves.

A school of dolphins now appears. As they are swimming along playfully, they begin to breach the water near the boat, splashing salty water onto the deck. You are now wet and laughing. You slip out of the boat and are now swimming among the carefree dolphins.

Any worries or concerns you have are fading away quickly as you immerse yourself totally into the fluidity of the ocean. You are filled with joy and peace, reveling in the moment. You are now floating on top of the water, looking up at the sky and basking in the feel of the sun on your skin. Ah, perfection.

Soon the dolphins swim away, into deeper waters. You are now swimming toward the shore. Within a few arm strokes, your feet touch the sand on the bottom. You stand upright and walk up onto the sandy beach.

You are now sitting in the wet sand near the water's edge. You are building a magnificent sandcastle. The tide begins to roll in and your beautiful sandcastle is being washed away. You are now lying upon the sand, allowing the tidal waters to flood over your body with their continuing waves.

As you are lying on the sand with the water rushing over you, you realize that you are a part of the sand. You realize you are a part of the water. You also realize you are a part of the air above you. You are aware that you are a part of everything and that you are no longer feeling as if you are a separate being. Not ever a separate being, you now know that you are always part of the whole.

PART 3

TREATMENT FUNDAMENTALS

*You have a treasure within you that is infinitely
greater than anything the world can offer.*

Eckhart Tolle

In this part, you'll journey further into your experience of the healing art of Reiki. You'll discover how to establish your own Reiki routine for self-treatments and find out why this is a crucial component of healing others with Reiki. You'll learn the basic hand placement techniques for performing Reiki. Then, you'll explore the ins and outs of treating others with Reiki, including how to establish good communication with the recipient, how to set boundaries, and what to expect when your energies blend with the recipient's. Next you'll learn about the power of Reiki symbols and how to participate in and arrange Reiki shares. Finally, you'll see how to treat physical aches and pains with Reiki.

CHAPTER 6

SELF-TREATMENTS

The most powerful relationship you will ever have is the relationship with yourself.

Steve Maraboli

PRACTICING REIKI THROUGH self-treatments helps to process and sustain the positive changes that an attunement to Reiki promises. When you are ill, self-treatments will help bring you back to good health. When you are healthy, self-treatments will reinforce your vitality and strengthen your immune system. Giving a Reiki self-treatment is easy—all you need are your hands, your body, and a willingness to heal and be healed.

A Regular Reiki Routine

Welcome Reiki into your life by making self-treatments a regular routine. Regularly practicing Reiki enhances other daily routines health-minded individuals incorporate into their lives—personal grooming, eating a healthy diet, practicing meditation, and exercising. It also helps boost your immune system and reduces feelings of stress and trauma.

Newly attuned Reiki Level I practitioners will benefit from doing full-body self-treatment sessions daily for the first four to six weeks. This helps you get better acquainted with practicing Reiki, and it also helps you become energetically and physically balanced. After those first weeks, you can switch to a regimen of one or two full-body self-treatments each week. How often you do Reiki self-treatments is entirely up to you. More is better than less, and less is better than none at all.

A Time Commitment

Please make time to carry out full treatments—you are worth it! Experiment by giving yourself treatments at different times to determine what hours of the day best suit your personal routine.

Early risers who do Reiki in the mornings have discovered that starting off their day with a treatment helps their day run more smoothly and harmoniously. Reiki helps them feel better equipped to confront their daily problems and deal with those life hurdles that get in their way from time to time.

REIKI REFLECTIONS

Our lifestyles do not always allow us the luxury of doing Reiki in a quiet or relaxing setting. Rather than forego Reiki altogether, it is better to do Reiki wherever you can, regardless of the environment. Reiki will work on the bus or the subway, and even in the middle of rush hour, if that's where you happen to be at the time it is called for.

Night owls, on the other hand, may mind getting up an hour earlier to perform a treatment. It could make them cranky and more tired.

If your body craves sleep, it will not be open to the idea of being awakened to apply Reiki. It seems self-defeating to forcibly awaken a slumbering body for the sake of applying a relaxation technique. Midmornings and afternoons are often the best times for Reiki if your workday allows either or both.

Doing self-treatments at bedtime can be a good option if you are experiencing insomnia or are sleep deprived, since Reiki can help lull you to sleep. However, a time when your body is already relaxing is probably not the most favorable time for a Reiki session, because Reiki's relaxing properties can put you to sleep before you've finished the treatment.

Think about your daily schedule and how you function best. Once you've established the time of day most conducive to your lifestyle, commit to doing your self-treatments until it becomes a regular habit.

Relaxing with Reiki

Preferably, Reiki treatments are done in solitude, either in quietness or with soft music being played in the background. Including Reiki self-treatments in an already hectic and time-squeezed schedule doesn't mean you have to sacrifice other activities that you enjoy. Your Reiki self-treatments can be incorporated into other relaxing practices that are already a part of your routine. Here are some ideas:

- Perform Reiki self-treatments while you are reclining on the couch watching television or listening to music.
- Integrate your meditation time with your Reiki treatment.
- Give yourself Reiki while soaking in a hot bubble bath.

Treat Trauma with Triple Treatments

Even the most balanced people have had their legs weaken and buckle out from under them when life throws them an unexpected curve ball and catches them off-guard. Job losses, deaths, divorces, accidents—all of these can flip a normally calm demeanor upside down. When impacted with a traumatic event, fight back by giving yourself three full-body Reiki treatments every day for three consecutive days.

After three days of self-Reiki sessions, reassess how you are doing, then ask yourself:

- Am I coping better?
- Am I sleeping adequately?
- Am I eating properly?
- Is my mind calm?
- Is my body centered?
- Am I able to breathe normally?

If your answer is no to any of these questions, continue beefing up your regular self-Reiki practice. Employing the help of another Reiki practitioner for treatment may be more effective in treating trauma than self-treating. Consider alternating self-treatments with receiving Reiki from another practitioner until you are feeling more in balance. Seeking help from a physician, energy medicine practitioner, or other qualified therapist, in addition to Reiki, may be necessary to fully address imbalances that occur when impacted by a traumatic event or enduring a stressful situation.

REIKI REFLECTIONS

If you feel that Reiki is not adequately treating your symptoms, it is okay, even advisable, to seek out other types of therapies. However, you do not have to choose between Reiki and another healing technique. Reiki is a team player; it complements all other therapies.

Preparing for a Full-Body Session

You don't need much to perform a full-body Reiki session on yourself. During the treatment, you can lie down on a bed, couch, reclining chair, or clean, carpeted floor. Just make certain that you're as comfortable as possible before and during treatment. A full-body Reiki treatment will take roughly sixty to ninety minutes to complete.

Make certain that the room you choose for your Reiki sessions is temperature controlled. It should be heated or cooled to match your personal comfort level. Keep a light wrap or blanket nearby with which to cover yourself in case you feel chilled at any time during the treatment. Reiki energies tend to produce heat, but influxes of both hot and cold temperatures can occur throughout the session. As the Reiki session progresses, you may be surprised to experience a change from the coolness of an air-conditioned room to an atmosphere of coziness and warmth.

Wash your hands thoroughly before you begin. You may want to remove any rings or bracelets from your fingers and wrists, especially if you are sensitive to the vibrational energies of gold, silver, or gemstones. When you place your hands on your body, be gentle, gentle, gentle! No pressure needs to be applied, since it is the exchange of ki energies that effectively does the healing work for you. When you place your hands, palms facing downward, onto your body, Reiki will begin to flow automatically. It is as simple as that.

When you use your hands to administer Reiki, hold the fingers and thumbs of each of your hands snugly together so there are no obvious gaps or spaces between them. Remember: all you need is a light touch to get the ki flowing. See Figure 6.1.

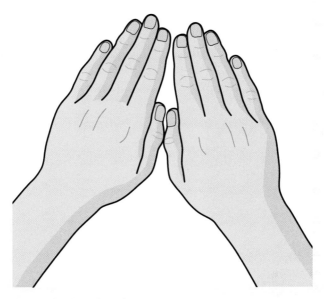

Figure 6.1 *Reiki hands*

Basic Hand Placements

The newly attuned Reiki Level I practitioner should carry out a precise sequence of hand placements during each full treatment. Always begin at the face placement and move downward. Devote five minutes to each placement in order to make sure you don't neglect any part of your body and so that each body part is given equal consideration. Wear a watch or place a clock within your visual range so that you can closely monitor the time spent on each placement.

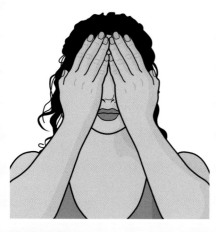

Figure 6.2
Placement 1: Face

Place the palms of your hands against the sides of your face, cupping your hands softly over your eyes. Rest the tips of your fingers gently against your forehead. Do not cover your nose and mouth—leave them exposed between your hands. Take care not to squeeze your nostrils, as you do not want to obstruct your breathing. Hold the fingers and thumbs of each of your hands snugly together so there are no obvious gaps or spaces between them. See Fig. 6.2.

Take your hands and place the base of each palm just slightly above your ears. Wrap both your palms and fingers along your skull, so that your fingertips meet at the crown. See Fig. 6.3.

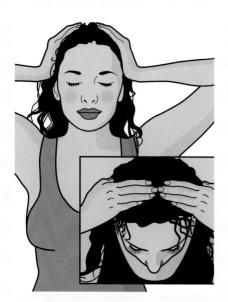

Figure 6.3
Placement 2: Crown and top of the head

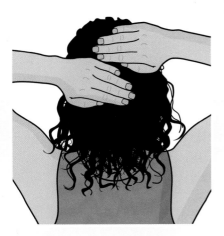

Cross your arms behind your head, placing one hand on the back of your head and the other directly below it and just above the nape of your neck. See Fig. 6.4.

Figure 6.4
Placement 3: Back of the head

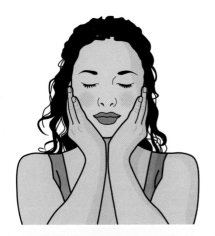

Cup your chin and jaw line in your hands, so that your inner wrists touch beneath your chin. Gently rest your fingertips over your earlobes. See Fig. 6.5.

Figure 6.5 *Placement 4: Chin and jaw line*

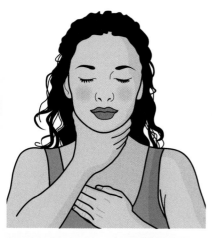

Place your right hand over the front of your neck, grasping your throat gently while allowing your neck to be held inside the space between your outward-extended thumb and fingers. Rest your left hand on top of your chest, between your collarbone and your heart. See Fig. 6.6.

Figure 6.6
Placement 5: Neck, collarbone, and heart

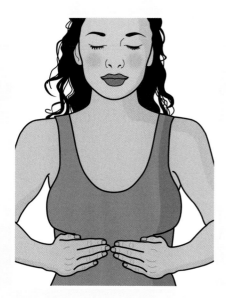

Place your hands on your rib cage, just below your breasts, with your fingertips touching. Your elbows should be bent back a little. See Fig. 6.7.

Figure 6.7
Placement 6: Ribs

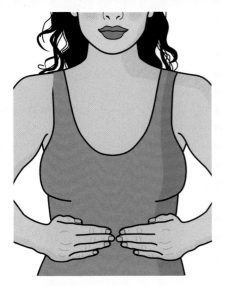

Place your hands on your solar plexus area, just above your navel. Keep your elbows bent and allow your fingertips to touch. See Fig. 6.8.

Figure 6.8
Placement 7: Abdomen

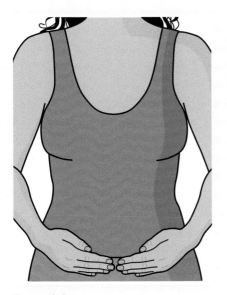

Place your right hand over your right pelvic bone and place your left hand over your left pelvic bone, so that your fingertips touch in the center. See Fig. 6.9.

Figure 6.9
Placement 8: Pelvic bones

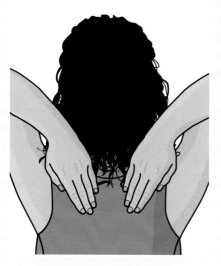

Reach over the top of your shoulders and place your hands on your shoulder blades. If you cannot reach your shoulder blades, reach only as far as you are able to comfortably. As an option, you can rest your hands on the tops of your shoulders. See Fig. 6.10.

Figure 6.10
Placement 9: Shoulders and shoulder blades

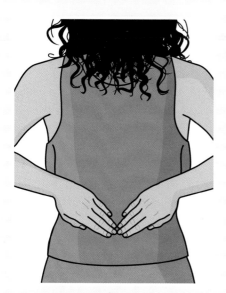

Reach behind your back, elbows bent, and place your hands on the middle of your back. Allow your fingertips to touch, if you are able to do so comfortably. See Fig. 6.11.

Figure 6.11
Placement 10: Midback

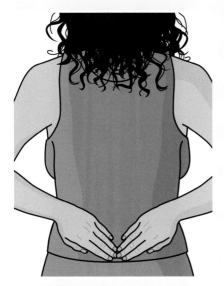

Reach behind your back, elbows bent, and place your hands on your lower back. Allow your fingertips to touch, if you are able to do so comfortably. See Fig. 6.12.

Figure 6.12
Placement 11: Lower back

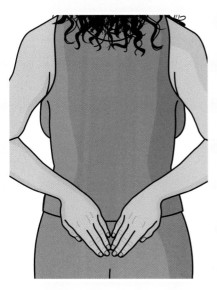

Reach behind your back, elbows bent, and place your hands on your sacral region. See Fig 6.13.

Figure 6.13
Placement 12: Sacrum

REIKI REFLECTIONS

Take your time and follow through with each placement that you are able to make. If you rush through Reiki's hand placements, you could very well be forfeiting the healing benefits of the hand placement set.

Traditional Usui Reiki Hand Placements

The Usui System of Natural Healing uses twelve basic hand placements in a full-body self-treatment. (In addition, there are other variations and alternative hand placements offered by nontraditional Reiki systems.) The twelve basic hand placements used in giving a full-body Reiki treatment include four placements on the head, four on the front of the body, and four placements on the back of the body.

Nontraditional Reiki Hand Placements

In addition to the twelve traditional Reiki hand placements for self-treatment, you may also add two others—the knee placement and the ankle-and-foot placement. To carry out the knee placement, place one hand over the top of your right knee and place your other hand underneath the same knee. Repeat this hand placement to treat your left knee.

The ankle-and-foot placement requires that you bend your knee in order for your hands to reach your ankle and foot comfortably. Place your left palm on the inside of your left foot, over the anklebone, fingers curled around the top of the foot. At the same time, grasp the sole of your right foot with your right hand. Reverse these hand placements to treat your left foot and right ankle.

Is It Okay to Skip Hand Placements?

Some people may complain that a particular placement is difficult to carry out or maintain for five minutes—for instance, the shoulder blades and back placements. If you cannot reach these areas, it is okay for you to skip them. The hand placements are taught as guidelines and are not set in stone. Reiki Level II practitioners can send distant Reiki to their own body parts that are unreachable.

Is It Working?

Each person will experience a Reiki session differently. Some people don't feel much of anything. If that's the case with you, keep in mind that just because you don't feel anything, it doesn't mean that nothing is happening. Trust that Reiki is working and continue to move through the different hand placements.

Other people will notice shifts of energies occurring. You may notice your palms are generating pulsing energies, or you may sense energy fluctuations pulsing through your entire body as it receives the ki vibrations.

It is normal for Reiki to flow better in some placements than in others, or, at times, to not flow at all. Anytime you feel as if the flow of Reiki is blocked, taking a few deep breaths can help start it flowing again.

REIKI REFLECTIONS

There is nothing sexual about touching yourself when applying Reiki. In applying self-treatments, it is perfectly acceptable to touch your breasts and genitalia. But it is not acceptable to touch someone else's private parts when you are treating him or her.

Interval Treatments

One way of dealing with a busy schedule is to make sure you do each of the twelve hand placements for at least five minutes at different intervals throughout the day. Map out your daily activities and combine them in partnership with the different hand placements so that they are done each day. Here is a sample schedule of interval treatments for all twelve hand placements:

- Placement 1, face: shortly after waking up in the morning and before getting out of bed
- Placement 2, crown and top of the head: in the morning, when you take a shower (you can do this placement as you stand in the hot streaming water)
- Placement 3, back of the head: while sitting at the breakfast table before or after you have your first meal of the day
- Placement 4, chin and jaw line: when you get into your car to drive to work or for errands, either before you start the engine or while the engine is warming up (after the session, you'll be able to drive to your workplace in a state of peace and tranquility)
- Placement 5, neck, collarbone, and heart: at lunchtime (if you are eating at a restaurant, you can do it after you've ordered and are waiting for your lunch to be served)
- Placement 6, ribs: mid-afternoon, while you are sitting at your desk or at the coffee break table
- Placement 7, abdomen: while sitting in the car before you drive home from your workplace
- Placement 8, pelvic bones: while you are sitting during your ten-minute meditation practice
- Placement 9, shoulders and shoulder blades: while sitting at the kitchen table prior to preparing your evening meal
- Placements 10, 11, and 12, midback, lower back, and sacrum: in the evening, either while you are reclining and watching television or while relaxing in your bed before going to sleep

Are You Avoiding Self-Treatments?

If you find yourself avoiding Reiki self-treatments, ask yourself why. People sometimes make excuses for not doing self-treatments because they, consciously or unconsciously, feel unworthy of love and healing. Perhaps they originally signed up to take a class and were attuned to Reiki because they wanted to have a means to extend love and healing to others. What these individuals have yet to fully comprehend is that in avoiding self-treatments, they are hindering their potential to help others.

Although Reiki practitioners are often referred to as healers, they are merely facilitators of healing energies. This means that you, in your role as a Reiki practitioner, have no power to heal others. Rather, you serve a supportive role, assisting another person in his healing journey. Ask yourself why you are willing to assist others in their journeys to heal but are reluctant to support your own journey toward wellness.

You may ask, "If giving Reiki to others helps them and also helps clear away blockages or congestion within my own body, why not skip self-treatments altogether?" But, never doing self-treatments and relying solely on treating others as a means to clear your own issues is not the most efficient or loving course of action to take when serving others. Purposely choosing not to do Reiki self-treatments and to give Reiki only to others is denying yourself deeper levels of active healing. The Reiki that flows through you while you are giving someone else a treatment is outwardly focused—after all, the intent is for Reiki to flow through you. Reiki will clear any blockages in your body that are obstructing the pathway to get to the other person, but it will not disperse into the deeper places that need healing within you.

Routinely doing self-treatments is fundamental to Reiki. A practitioner will become more and more comfortable with her whole being each time the Reiki hand placements are applied during full-body self-treatments.

When used to treat others, Reiki's role is a passive one; whereas in applying self-treatments, Reiki takes on a more active role. Routinely doing self-treatments will help keep your ki passageways free of any impurities or negative energy that accumulates in your body from day to day and will also allow Reiki to penetrate more deeply into your body to negate any imbalances. Regular self-treatment practices will also allow you to assist others in a more loving and balanced manner when you, in turn, give Reiki to them.

CHAPTER 7

TREATING OTHERS

*Throughout history, "tender loving care"
has uniformly been recognized as a
valuable element in healing.*

Larry Dossey

IN THIS CHAPTER, you'll have the chance to explore how to give Reiki treatments to others. Open communication between the Reiki practitioner and the recipient is extremely important, and here you'll receive pointers on how best to accomplish this. When the practitioner and recipient agree to team up as giver and receiver of healing, the two individuals form a special bond, a sort of contractual relationship. That relationship may require you to set boundaries—an important topic covered here. While the individual roles of practitioner and recipient may be played out very differently, the primary goal—to promote relaxation and well-being—remains essentially the same. In this chapter, you'll discover how to deliver Reiki treatments to a wide variety of recipients.

Newly Attuned Exuberance

As a newly attuned Reiki practitioner, you may be very anxious to jump in and get busy giving Reiki to everyone. However, your exuberance may be met with varying degrees of apprehension from friends and family members. Try not to be overzealous in selling the benefits of Reiki. Offer to give Reiki treatments to your friends so they can experience it for themselves, but don't be surprised if your offers are politely rejected. Some people are simply not as open to Reiki as others. It may take a while for them to warm up to the idea. Respect their feelings and don't push.

No Guinea Pigs

Once you've identified and confirmed a few people among your circle of family and friends who are willing to allow you to give them a full-body Reiki treatment, be careful not to give them the impression that they're serving as guinea pigs in your Reiki experiments. You also shouldn't imply in any way that you are unsure of your effectiveness in applying Reiki. Certainly, you are new at this, but Reiki will flow proficiently, regardless of those through whom it will flow. Is the measure of a gallon of water any less when it is poured out of a brand-new plastic jug than when it is poured from an aged clay pitcher? Of course not. The same is true of the flow of Reiki. Reiki will flow at the appropriate levels as needed by the Reiki recipient, whether or not the practitioner is a beginner or a more advanced channeler of Reiki.

Practicing Reiki in Varying Capacities

Naturally, your awareness of how Reiki works and your confidence in using Reiki will improve over time. Moreover, as you give more treatments, you will come to decide in what way being a Reiki practitioner best serves you. Some Reiki practitioners are content in doing only self-treatments, while others are also interested in sharing Reiki among immediate family members and their closest friends and relatives. Still other practitioners are drawn to becoming full-time healers and making their healing practice an integral part of their livelihood.

Pretreatment Communication

It is your responsibility to help the recipient feel comfortable and reassured before the treatments begin. Be friendly and welcoming. Do your best to address any feelings of anxiety, confusion, or uncertainty that are expressed, either verbally or through body language, and attempt to answer fully all questions that arise.

It is normal for a person who meets with a Reiki practitioner for the first time to feel a variety of emotions. Among these emotions are excitement, apprehension, expectation, and nervousness. Having someone touch your body, even in a healing atmosphere, can feel like an intrusion of your personal space. Because of this, it is important that the practitioner take some time to help the recipient feel more at ease and establish a level of trust.

Go Over the Treatment Step by Step

Carefully explain the treatment process, delineating exactly what will take place. Naturally, you will not know what your recipient's specific experience may be, as everyone greets Reiki differently. However, you can give an outline of the basic steps that will take place. Here is a list of points you can share with the Reiki recipient before the session begins:

- Approximately how long the treatment will take (sixty to ninety minutes)
- What the recipient needs to do during the treatment (lie on her back for the first part of the treatment and on her stomach for the second part of the treatment)
- How the Reiki recipient will need to be dressed (fully clothed, except for her shoes and belt; loose-fitting attire is preferable)
- Whether it's okay for the recipient to talk, be silent, or even fall asleep during the treatment (it is)
- How you will touch the recipient's body with your hands during the session (describe the hand placements and explain that you will begin with the face and move downward)
- How to breathe during the treatment (explain that you may ask her to take some breaths from time to time to help the Reiki flow more evenly or to help release blockages)
- What happens at the end of the treatment (you will comb through the recipient's aura to clear it of stagnant energies that were released from her body)
- What to do in the next twenty-four hours (take care of themselves by eating well, drinking water, and allowing their body to physically or emotionally release any energy that is no longer serving them)

After explaining the treatment step by step, be prepared to answer any additional questions the recipient might have about Reiki and your methodology.

Setting Intentions

Pretreatment communication creates a nurturing atmosphere for healing to occur during a Reiki treatment. Furthermore, it helps ensure you and the recipient are "on the same page" in regard to what will become the focus of the treatment.

Here are a few questions you could ask the recipient to help you both discover a suitable healing intention to use for the treatment:

- How are you feeling today?
- What are your physical health concerns?
- How is your current mood?
- Is anything disturbing you?
- What are your expectations for this treatment?
- Do you want to make changes in your perceptions?
- What pushes your emotional buttons?
- What are your current and most troublesome fears?
- Do you have normal sleep patterns?
- Are you an excessive worrier?

These and other similar questions can help pinpoint a specific focus for the Reiki treatment. Prompting the recipient to state her intention out loud prior to the treatment can be very effective in helping the focus and flow of Reiki.

REIKI REFLECTIONS

Reiki practitioners have no legal right to diagnose conditions and should not refer to the people they are treating as patients. However, you can urge clients to seek medical advice from a licensed physician regarding symptoms or conditions that you intuit during treatment. It is a good idea to have a list of physicians, therapists, and other holistic practitioners handy so you can refer your clients to them.

Hand Placements for Treating Others

The hand placements for giving a Reiki treatment are much like those used for self-treatment. In treating another person, begin at the face placement, complete the other head placements, and move down the body. Allow approximately three to five minutes per hand placement. A full-body treatment for another person normally lasts from sixty to ninety minutes, just as a self-treatment does. The hand placements are only guidelines. As you become more proficient, you will learn to place and move your hands intuitively.

The First Four Hand Placements

Begin the Reiki treatment with the person lying on his back. Perform Gassho and state the healing intention that was decided on during pretreatment communication. Sit down in a chair directly behind the recipient's head.

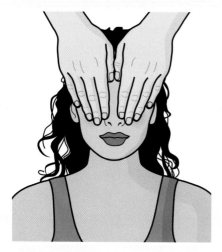

Position your hands over the sides of the recipient's face, cupping your fingers lightly over the eyes and placing the palms of your hands gently upon the recipient's forehead. Do not cover the recipient's nose and mouth. Be careful not to squeeze the nostrils—you do not want to obstruct the recipient's breathing. See Fig. 7.1.

Figure 7.1
Placement 1: Face

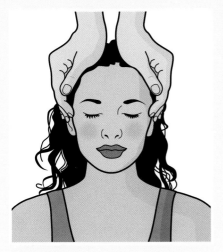

Place the base of your palms, inner wrists touching, on top of the recipient's head at the crown. Wrap your palms and fingers around the recipient's skull, allowing your fingertips to touch the tops of her ears. See Fig. 7.2.

Figure 7.2
Placement 2: Crown and top of the head

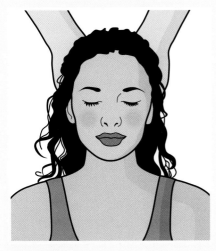

Slip your hands gently underneath the recipient's head, forming a cradle for the head. Rest the back of your hands on the massage table. See Fig. 7.3.

Figure 7.3
Placement 3: Back of the head

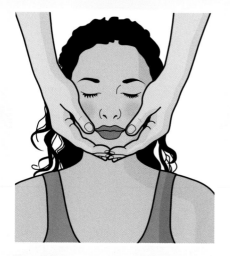

Mold your hands gently around the recipient's jaw line, so that your fingertips are touching under the recipient's chin and the heels of your hands are resting beneath his ears or over his earlobes. See Fig. 7.4.

Figure 7.4
Placement 4: Chin and jaw line

Switch Positions for the Next Placement

Placement 5 can be done either while sitting directly behind the recipient's head or sitting at the recipient's side. Choosing where to sit while applying this placement depends on the length of your arms. If your arms are not long enough to comfortably reach the recipient's throat and heart while sitting behind the recipient's head, try moving your chair closer to the side of the table.

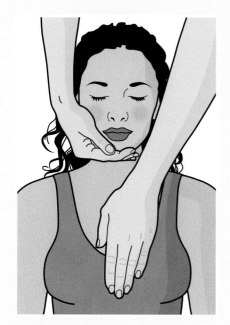

Wrap your right hand around the recipient's neck, allowing the right side of the neck to be held inside the space between your outward-extended thumb and fingers. Alternatively, allow your right hand to hover over the neck. This option is used when the person you are treating feels uneasy about your hand actually touching her throat. Stretch your left arm out and place your left hand over the recipient's heart. See Fig. 7.5.

Figure 7.5
Placement 5: Neck, collarbone, and heart

REIKI REFLECTIONS

Be especially careful not to aggravate the recipient by doing a hand placement that might cause sudden pain, stress, or any degree of discomfort. The throat is a sensitive area that many people do not like to have touched because of fears of strangulation or suffocation. Always be sensitive to thoughts and feelings the Reiki recipient might harbor.

The Next Three Hand Placements

Hand placements 6, 7, and 8 are employed while you are sitting either to the left or right of the recipient; it does not matter which side you choose. Move your chair alongside the recipient's body as needed. Using a swivel chair on wheels works especially well for this purpose.

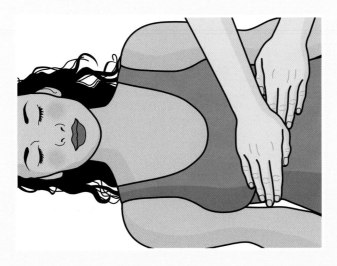

Figure 7.6
Placement 6:
Ribs

Place your hands on the recipient's rib cage, just below the recipient's breasts. See Fig. 7.6.

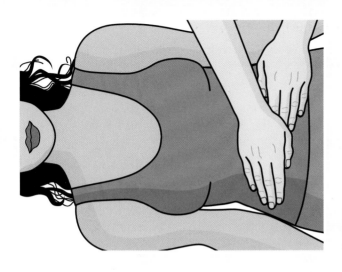

Figure 7.7
Placement 7:
Abdomen

Place your hands on the solar plexus area, just above the recipient's navel. See Fig. 7.7.

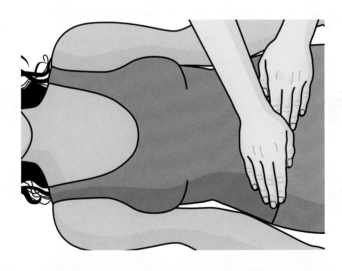

Figure 7.8
Placement 8:
Pelvic bones

Place one hand over each of the recipient's pelvic bones. See Fig. 7.8.

The Last Four Hand Placements

These final hand placements are done while the recipient is lying on his stomach. The practitioner can remain at either side of the recipient. It is likely that the recipient will be very relaxed, even sleepy, from the Reiki being applied thus far. If necessary, assist the recipient in making the adjustment from lying on his back to lying on his stomach. Attach the face rest to your massage table and assist the recipient in placing his face down. Use a soft cloth-fitted cover, handkerchiefs, or a few facial tissues to cover the face rest, but be sure to leave the center hole open for breathing.

REIKI REFLECTIONS

The shoulders are an area of a person's body where you will often sense concentrated amounts of pent-up energy. This is because emotional burdens and worrisome feelings are often stored there. When you are giving a full-body Reiki treatment, spend a few extra minutes on this area.

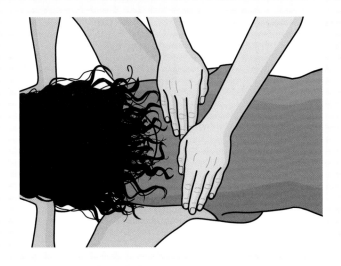

Figure 7.9
Placement 9:
Shoulder blades

Place your hands on the recipient's shoulder blades. See Fig. 7.9.

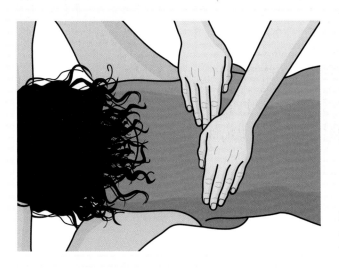

Figure 7.10
Placement 10:
Midback

Place your hands on the middle of the recipient's back.
See Fig. 7.10.

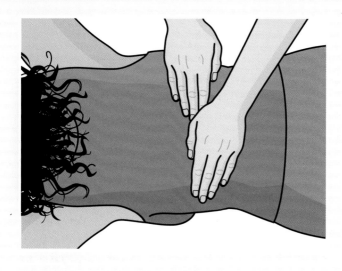

Figure 7.11
Placement 11:
Lower back

Place your hands on the recipient's lower back. See. Fig. 7.11.

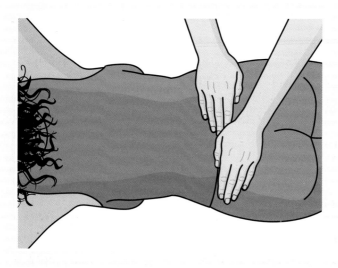

Figure 7.12
Placement 12:
Sacrum

Place your hands on the recipient's sacral region. See Fig. 7.12.

Blending of Personal Energies

Any time we are within a few feet of another person, our auras blend together and a fusion of energy takes place. This, in turn, can create a mixed bag of emotions and sensations. Depending on the circumstances and the relationships between you and the other person, the feelings that surface from energy fusion can range anywhere from pleasingly desirable to fearfully intrusive.

It is often difficult for most of us to share close quarters with total strangers. Consider how you feel when you are in close proximity to a stranger when riding in an elevator or sitting next to a stranger at the movie theater. Most people's auras will shrink closer to their physical bodies as they try to maintain energetic boundaries. During a Reiki session, the auras of the practitioner and recipient will naturally blend. The practitioner not only sits near the recipient, but she actually reaches out and touches the recipient's body.

Clearing Auras

At the end of the session, the Reiki practitioner combs the recipient's aura to clear it of any energetic debris that has lifted from the physical body during the treatment by moving the hands in multiple circular motions or using feathering sweeps of the hands over the body. As the aura is cleansed, a request is silently made for the negative energies to be transformed into positive ones, to be used for universal goodness.

Reiki Energy versus Personal Energy

Reiki is a universal source of energy that flows through the practitioner and into the recipient. Personal energies are not being transferred or exchanged. To be clear—the practitioner is not giving away any of his own energy to the recipient, nor is the recipient taking energy away from the practitioner.

The fusion of personal energies during treatment can feel as if it is part of Reiki, but that isn't actually the case. The blending of personal energies happens as a consequence of the practitioner and recipient being near each other. Energy fusion experiences can be magnified when individuals empathetically tune in to these personal energies. The personal energy fusion between the practitioner and recipient during a Reiki treatment can be difficult to distinguish from the energy flow of Reiki until you begin to recognize that Reiki has no emotional charge or flavoring.

If Reiki energy were a drink, it would have no taste and could be described as filtered water with no impurities. If personal energies were beverages, they would have distinctive flavors such as sugary colas, pulpy juices, and chocolate milk.

Creating Boundaries

As word spreads within your community that you are a Reiki practitioner, you may find yourself inundated with requests to give Reiki treatments. You may find yourself being asked to give Reiki treatments to your neighbors, relatives, friends, friends of friends, relatives of friends, friends of relatives, and occasionally even pets of your relatives' friends! Yes, you read that right.

It is very important to set clear boundaries and figure out whom you are willing to treat and when you are willing to treat them. You have every right to refuse treatment to anyone without justifying your feelings. Certainly, it is unreasonable to give Reiki to people whom you feel are not suitably receptive to it, but it is equally unreasonable for you to feel required to give Reiki every time it is requested of you.

If you ever feel pressured or uneasy when asked to give Reiki to someone, it is a good idea to take some time to evaluate your feelings before agreeing to it. Anytime you feel strongly that you do not want to give a Reiki treatment to someone, embrace those feelings without hesitation and politely refuse. Reiki, when done under pressured circumstances, is unlikely to result in a positive outcome. It is crucial that the people being treated want the treatment for their own healing journey and not merely to please a friend or relative who thinks they would benefit from Reiki.

Basic Hand Placements for Seated Reiki

If you are working on a client who can't lie down for a long period of time, can only sit for a short time, or needs to use a wheelchair, Reiki can be done while in a shortened, seated session. Before you begin the placements, instruct the recipient to take a few deep, relaxing breaths, and take a few deep, cleansing breaths of your own.

Here are the basic hand placements that may be used for carrying out a shortened Reiki treatment when a person is sitting upright. Hold each position for two to five minutes.

1. Shoulder Position—While standing directly behind the recipient, place your hands on both of his shoulders.
2. Crown Position—Place your palms on the top of the recipient's head.
3. Forehead Position—Move to the recipient's side. Place one hand on the area between the back of the head and the top of the spine. Place your other hand on his forehead.
4. Throat Position—Place one hand on the recipient's seventh protruding cervical vertebra. Place your other hand directly in front of the pit of his throat.
5. Breastbone Position—Place one hand on the recipient's breastbone and the other hand on the recipient's back, in the same area opposite the breastbone.

6. Stomach Position—Place one hand on the recipient's solar plexus and the other hand on the back region opposite his solar plexus.
7. Pelvic Position—Place one hand on the recipient's front pelvic region and the other hand on the back pelvic region.

Finish the session with an aura sweeping to clear any debris lingering in the auric field of the recipient's body. This should take approximately one minute.

Reiki Treatments at Healthcare Facilities

In giving Reiki treatments to patients in hospitals, clinics, and nursing homes, it is important that you do not interfere with any of the facility's rules and routines. Check in with the staff to make sure that your presence and timing of a Reiki treatment for a patient will not interfere with meal times, scheduled lab tests, family visiting hours, and so on, and will not interfere with any of the patient's prescribed medical treatments or restrictions, such as limited movement. Be sure that the staff understands what giving a Reiki treatment to a patient under their care will entail.

When paying a home visit, it is helpful to bring along a portable massage table to use during the Reiki treatments. However, bringing along your Reiki table is not usually feasible in hospital rooms, since space is limited and will not accommodate a table. There may also be liability issues or hospital rules against the use of equipment not owned by the facility.

If the recipient is confined to a hospital bed, do the best you can to apply all the Reiki hand placements without causing any discomfort to the patient or to yourself. Eliminate any hand placements that you cannot perform easily. If the recipient is not bedfast, you can ask her to sit upright in a bedside chair or lie down in the hospital bed with her head at the foot of the bed in order for you to do the Reiki head placements.

Whether giving Reiki to family members, friends, or clients, giving full-body treatments to others involves time and effort. Reiki will do its job without exhaustion. However, practitioners should remember to honor their own needs first so as not to overspend their personal energies.

Caregiving and Reiki

The caregivers in our medical communities include doctors, chiropractors, nurses, counselors, therapists, nursing home aides, and hospice workers. However, the title of "caregiver" also applies to individuals who personally assist their relatives and friends who are aged, ailing, or indisposed. Parents are caregivers as well—they provide care for their kids. All Reiki practitioners are caregivers in the sense that they give of themselves when caring for others with Reiki treatments.

REIKI REFLECTIONS

Reiki will treat numerous physical maladies, emotional imbalances, and spiritual afflictions. Reiki will also extend its healing energies to nurture your environment and strengthen your relationships.

Caregivers are at high risk of physical and emotional burnout. Taking care of another person, especially if his needs are considerable, can result in a great expenditure of one's physical and emotional energy. Therefore, it is vital that the caregiver's depleted energies are replenished. Fortunately, caregivers can rely on Reiki not only by giving treatments to their charges, but also by carrying out self-treatments to keep themselves energized and balanced.

Reiki Benefits Everyone

Reiki's gift of increased energy and vitality can be extended to anyone. It doesn't matter what a person's gender, race, intelligence level, or financial status is. Reiki is not a healing energy reserved only for the elite, wealthy, educated, or spiritually evolved. Reiki is free to anyone who wants it. It does not cost anything but a little of your time.

Treating Root Causes

Because Reiki flows to where it is needed, its natural course is to first deal with any apparent symptoms of illness or dis-ease. When Reiki treatments are discontinued after your symptoms have diminished or been eliminated, don't be surprised if these conditions recur. Reiki will only serve as a Band-Aid if you abandon its use too hastily. Through consistent and continued use of Reiki, the root cause of any given illness can be treated. It is when the root cause is treated fully that Reiki can be called a "cure."

Benefits of Reiki

The list of benefits that Reiki offers is comprehensive. Basically, Reiki will benefit you by empowering you whenever you feel weakened or downtrodden. Here is a list of some of the specific benefits Reiki offers:

- Reiki's calming effects can reduce our anxieties.
- It may go to the core of imbalances embedded within our bodies to bring about balance.
- Pain, stresses, and agitations that are associated with long-term suffering can benefit from cumulative Reiki treatments.
- Reiki can be safely used in conjunction with all other conventional health practices.
- Reiki offers the kind of energetic vitality that can spark our innate creativity.
- Reiki's ability to awaken and sharpen our psychic perceptions heightens awareness of our dreams.

- Blessing our food and drinks with Reiki before consuming them will vitalize and purify them.
- Reiki's gentle energies are conducive to comforting anyone who is suffering from grief. It helps the grief process run its course in a calmer or less painful way.
- Reiki tames discord and trouble, bringing harmony to the recipient or situation that is out of sync.
- The swiftness of Reiki's healing properties has demonstrated that it is an effective complementary first-aid treatment for injuries, although it shouldn't be used on a fresh break of a bone.
- Reiki will treat emotional wounds and memories that are hurting our inner child.
- Reiki assists us in letting go of the aspects within our lives that negatively impact us.
- The manifesting facets of Reiki help to bring our intentions and goals to fruition.
- Reiki can expedite the body's natural healing ability, reducing the recovery periods that follow surgeries and injuries.
- Reiki's relaxing energies can induce sleep and relieve insomnia.
- Using Reiki may awaken or improve spiritual awareness.
- Reiki clears our bodies of impurities and stagnant energies.
- Reiki will penetrate beyond obvious systemic conditions of the body and treat the underlying causes of illness.
- Reiki can help you deal with special situations in your life, such as exams, job interviews, divorce, career changes, and family illness.

This list could be expanded for several more pages; there is simply no limit to the benefits that Reiki can bestow on those who are receptive to it. All of us can benefit from it—and so can our children, our parents and grandparents, and our animal companions. Even skeptical-minded individuals who look cautiously at Reiki can benefit from it if they are willing to explore its possibilities.

CHAPTER 8

ABSENTIA TREATMENTS

Wherever there is a human being, there is an opportunity for kindness.

Seneca

ABSENTIA REIKI TREATMENTS can be given to individuals who are not in physical contact with you. Similar to offering prayers, sending Reiki's healing energies in absentia (sometimes called remote or distance healing) involves visualization and mental focus, and it is done as a request for improvement in the recipient's health, life circumstance, and so on. In this chapter, you'll learn how best to give Reiki treatments when you're not physically able to perform them. But remember, absentia treatments are not a substitute for hands-on treatments; they are a convenient alternative for circumstances in which it is either impractical or simply not possible to do a hands-on treatment. But to use Reiki in absentia to its full effect you'll need to understand the importance of Reiki symbols, so let's begin with those.

The Power of Reiki Symbols

In order to execute remote healing, the Reiki practitioner must rely on the Reiki symbols, which were derived from written characters in the Japanese language. Students learn the first three Reiki symbols when they progress to Reiki Level II. These are the Power symbol, the Connection symbol, and the Harmony symbol. The remaining two symbols, the Master symbol and the Raku, are passed on to the Reiki Level III teacher to utilize in the attunement process when initiating new students to Reiki. The combined function of these symbols is to give Reiki practitioners focal points for their healing intentions.

REIKI REFLECTIONS

Reiki symbols are considered sacred and were kept secret for many generations among Reiki practitioners. Even today, many practitioners honor the tradition of keeping them hidden from view by never drawing them on paper and visualizing them from memory alone.

In addition to their use in distance healing, Reiki symbols are used in the attunement process and for directing, focusing, and increasing the flow of Reiki during hands-on healing. Reiki Level II students are taught how to draw and visualize the Reiki symbols to use in increasing power and focus of hands-on healing.

Working with the Symbols

The more you work with the symbols, the more familiar you will become with how each symbol has its own unique purposes. Learning about Reiki symbols goes far beyond any basic grasp of techniques you could be taught in a class or read in a book. You must use symbols when doing treatments to achieve that better understanding. By experimenting with them over a period of time, you will instinctively begin to appreciate how powerfully expansive and fluid these symbols are.

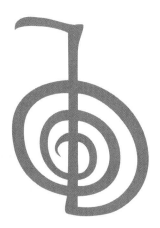

Figure 8.1 *Power symbol*

The Power Symbol

The first Reiki symbol, Cho Ku Rei, is the Power symbol. It is a spiral-shaped symbol that is often referred to as the light switch. The Cho Ku Rei symbol represents the engine that gives Reiki its initial boost. Whenever Reiki needs a nudge to get started or there is a need for an increase in power when applying Reiki, this symbol can be used. In absentia treatments, the Cho Ku Rei serves as the delivery system. See Fig. 8.1.

The Harmony Symbol

The second Reiki symbol, Sei Hei Ki, is the Harmony symbol. The Harmony symbol resembles a dragon. Its purpose is to promote the balance and harmony needed to heal our mental and emotional bodies. This symbol can be used in absentia treatments but isn't always needed. It is also known as the Protection symbol. See Fig. 8.2.

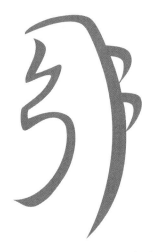

Figure 8.2 *Harmony symbol*

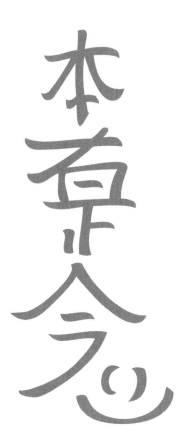

The Connection Symbol

The third Reiki symbol, Hon Sha Ze Sho Nen, is the Connection symbol. This symbol resembles a pagoda. Its primary purpose is to be used in transmitting absentia treatments. It also serves as a key to unlock information that is kept in the Akashic Records. See Fig. 8.3.

Traveling through past, present, and future events, this symbol defies time and space. The Hon Sha Ze Sho Nen is also an excellent tool to use in healings that focus on childhood traumas, inner-child therapy, and past-life issues.

Figure 8.3 *Connection symbol*

REIKI REFLECTIONS

The Akashic Records, also known as The Book of Life, may be described as the vibrational volumes where every experience (thought, action, and emotion) of every soul in existence is recorded. It is the "database" that psychics explore to glean prophetic and past-life information.

Master and Raku Symbols

The Master symbol, Dai Ko Myo, is used in both hands-on and absentia treatments by Reiki practitioners attuned to the Master Level. The essence of the Master symbol is love. It is considered the most powerful of all the symbols.

The Raku is used only in the attunement process when initiating practitioners into the different levels of Reiki. See Fig. 8.4 and 8.5.

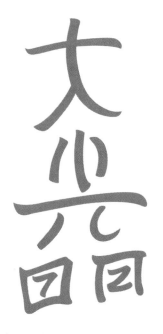

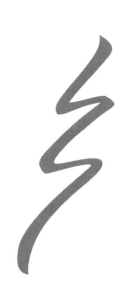

Figure 8.4 *Master symbol*   **Figure 8.5** *Raku symbol*

The Absentia Healing Formula

The following is a basic formula that uses three Reiki symbols known by Reiki Level II practitioners to begin an absentia Reiki treatment.

1. Draw a Cho Ku Rei symbol for power. As you draw the Power symbol, repeat the symbol's name three times: Cho Ku Rei, Cho Ku Rei, Cho Ku Rei.

2. Draw a Hon Sha Ze Sho Nen symbol for connection. As you draw the Connection symbol, repeat its name three times: Hon Sha Ze Sho Nen, Hon Sha Ze Sho Nen, Hon Sha Ze Sho Nen.

3. Make your Reiki request. State your healing intention, including the name and general location of the person to receive the absentia treatment.

4. Draw a Cho Ku Rei symbol. As you draw the Power symbol, say it three times: Cho Ku Rei, Cho Ku Rei, Cho Ku Rei.

5. Draw a Sei Hei Ki symbol for harmony. As you draw the Harmony symbol, say it three times: Sei Hei Ki, Sei Hei Ki, Sei Hei Ki.

6. Draw a Cho Ku Rei symbol. As you draw the Power symbol, say it three times: Cho Ku Rei, Cho Ku Rei, Cho Ku Rei.

Drawing a symbol does not necessarily mean actually drawing it on paper. Although rendering symbols on paper with ink can be very powerful, it is not always practical. You can draw them with your hands in the air and place the air-drawn symbols into objects or draw them mentally by visualizing them in your mind.

By drawing the symbols, you are bringing them into the open so that they are accessible in the physical world. By exposing them in this way, you are making their potential powers and purposes available to the Reiki recipient.

When drawing symbols in the air to be incorporated in absentia treatments, it is essential that each symbol be drawn completely before it is sent mentally. Symbols sent in fragments will not deliver the highest healing powers that whole symbols will.

Reiki Flash Cards

The absentia healing formula is sometimes taught in a Reiki class through the use of flash cards as instructional aides. Making your own set of Reiki flash cards is fun and easy. Only a few inexpensive materials are needed: blank index cards, a felt-tip marker, a pen or pencil, and one envelope. A complete set of flash cards for sending absentia Reiki to one individual will include:

- Three index cards with the Cho Ku Rei symbol drawn on them
- One index card with the Hon Sha Ze Sho Nen symbol drawn on it
- One index card with the Sei Hei Ki symbol drawn on it
- One blank index card

Use the felt-tip marker to draw the Reiki symbols on the cards. When incorporating flash cards as your focus, you stack the index cards face up, one on top of another, as you apply the absentia healing formula. Start with a Cho Ku Rei card on the bottom, then place the Hon Sha Ze Sho Nen card on top. Next, using a pen or pencil, write the name of the recipient and your intention statement on a blank index card. Place this request card on top of the Hon Sha Ze Sho Nen card. On top of the request card, you next place a second Cho Ku Rei card, followed by the Sei Hei Ki card. Last, place the final Cho Ku Rei card on top of the stack and place all six stacked cards inside a small envelope. Hold the envelope between your hands to allow the Reiki to flow to the recipient. To send Reiki to more than one recipient, simply include another request card and another Cho Ku Rei card for each additional person. As an option, you can include photographs of the recipients along with the Reiki flash cards inside the envelope.

Directing the Flow

Intention is the means through which Reiki is directed in doing either hands-on or absentia treatments. When giving a hands-on treatment, your primary intention as a practitioner is to facilitate a healing. This intention need not be stated since it is implied when your hands are placed on the body. Reiki will automatically flow to wherever it is needed, with no mental involvement of either the practitioner or the recipient. However, when mental intention is used, a linear pathway is opened. This cleared route allows Reiki to flow more effectively to the part of the body where attention is desired.

Direction is very important when facilitating an absentia healing. Through the use of mental focus, along with the Reiki symbols, Reiki's subtle healing energies can be directed to take a particular path. The practitioner is not controlling Reiki by using the symbols and using her mental powers. The practitioner who uses intent is still serving as Reiki's conduit, but with her concentrated involvement, the Reiki will travel more swiftly to the recipient, the main focus of the Reiki energies.

Obtaining Consent

Consent is always a determining factor in giving a Reiki treatment, regardless of whether or not it is carried out in absentia or in person. If your offer to give a hands-on treatment has been rejected, trying to override that person's decision to refuse Reiki by pursuing the route of an absentia treatment would be misguided. Ignoring a person's right to refuse is a deceptive maneuver and damages your integrity as a healer.

When Consent Cannot Be Obtained
However, there are a few acceptable circumstances in which you can send Reiki without being given verbal permission by the recipient:

1. The recipient is comatose or is for some other reason incapable of conveying his consent.
2. The parent of a young child has requested that you send Reiki to his son or daughter.

In Case of Recipient Resistance
It is acceptable for the Reiki practitioner to make an introductory statement of intention in order to indicate that Reiki will become available to the recipient only if she is willing to consent to it on a conscious or spiritual level. If you make such a statement, be sure to say that if the recipient declines Reiki, its healing energies will be made available for someone else who is willing to accept them. Some practitioners request that any excess Reiki energies from their absentia sendings be directed to the earth and used for positive global healing.

It is possible for a practitioner who is adept at perceiving the flow of Reiki to feel resistance from the recipient when sending absentia healing energies. Whenever you sense that the Reiki energy is not being welcomed by the recipient, the most appropriate action to take is to discontinue the treatment altogether. Never attempt to force Reiki on anyone who seems inclined to refuse it. To do so suggests that the practitioner is driven by ego, and this is unethical. Never assume that you, as a Reiki practitioner, know what is best for another person.

A More Mindful Approach

For some practitioners, giving an absentia treatment can be inherently more profound than doing a hands-on treatment. This is because possible distractions associated with being in direct contact with the other person's physical body and personality are removed.

When practitioners give hands-on treatments, their perception can be lessened because of people's chatter, masking abilities, body language, and many other factors, thus obstructing a keener awareness. Basically, we are confronted with the storefront dressings of the recipients we treat. Astral connections circumvent any exterior façade that clouds our perceptions when we are in physical contact with others, making our association with them less encumbered with purposeless information.

REIKI REFLECTIONS

It is common practice among Reiki practitioners to give an absentia treatment to a person the evening before the scheduled hands-on treatment. Doing this kind of preliminary healing helps ready the recipient's receptivity to Reiki's energies and often predetermines a more profound hands-on healing session.

When you are asked by someone to send absentia Reiki, you are being invited into that person's sacred space. Be respectful during your treatment, since the recipient is making herself vulnerable to your perceptions. This is not the time or place to play the role of an investigator, seeking to discover what secrets might be exposed by psychologically touring the recipient's personal energy field. Be mindful that confidentiality still applies.

Absentia Treatment Positions

Absentia Reiki treatments can last as long as full-body hands-on treatments. Find a comfortable chair to sit in while you are giving the distance treatment. An overstuffed chair or recliner works well. During the treatment you will be using your knees, thighs, and hips as spots for placing your hands. To apply the hand placements, imagine a miniature of the recipient lying on his back on your left leg and a miniature of the person lying on his stomach on your right leg. Before you apply your hands, bring forth the Reiki symbols and state your intention as outlined in the absentia healing formula.

Self As Surrogate

Here are the specific hand placements used in absentia treatments:

- Your left knee represents the recipient's face, crown, neck, and jaw line.
- Your left middle-thigh area represents the recipient's heart and upper chest.
- Your left upper-thigh area represents the recipient's ribs and abdomen.
- Your left hip area represents the recipient's pelvic bones.
- Your right knee represents the back of the recipient's head and his neck/throat area.
- Your right middle-thigh area represents the recipient's shoulder blades.
- Your right upper-thigh area represents the recipient's midback and lower-back regions.
- Your right hip area represents the recipient's sacral region.

Apply your hands to these placements on your lap in the same manner with which you would give a full-body treatment to a recipient who was actually in your presence. Allow three to five minutes per hand placement.

Teddy Bear Surrogates

A favorite way to send distance Reiki is by using a teddy bear as a surrogate. Choose a bear that fits comfortably on your lap. With an open hand, draw the Reiki symbols in the air and gently push them with your hand into the head or tummy of the bear as you state your intention for the absentia treatment. Proceed with the Reiki hand placements on the bear in the same manner you would on the recipient if he were actually present. You can finish the treatment by hugging the bear as a demonstration of your love being extended to the recipient.

Sending Reiki to a Group

Absentia Reiki can be sent to more than one individual at the same time. The Reiki energies received by the recipients are not lessened as a result of Reiki being dispensed to several people. Each person or group named in the practitioner's intention statement can benefit from the healing energies being offered. You may consider sending Reiki to particular groups of people or even to places or causes:

- Reiki can be sent to general cross-section groups such as farmers, teachers, newborns, and firefighters.
- Reiki can be sent to care organizations such as the Red Cross, UNICEF, the Salvation Army, or Habitat for Humanity.
- Reiki can be sent for special causes such as asking for survival of endangered animals, food for the hungry, homes for the homeless, and prosperity for the poor.
- Reiki can be sent to specific health advocate groups such as hospice caregivers, incest victims, and cancer survivors.
- Reiki can be sent to locations such as hospitals, schools, and prisons.

REIKI REFLECTIONS

Doing multiple healings at once clouds the practitioner's perception of how and where the Reiki is flowing. However, it is not always relevant that the practitioner be involved in how the Reiki energy is being used. Serving as a conduit for Reiki to be dispensed for the greater good of all concerned is always gratifying.

Many practitioners make sending absentia Reiki a part of their daily routines, much like a daily meditation practice. They will spend twenty to sixty minutes mindfully sending Reiki out to whoever is in need. You can create a special place in your home where you gather up photographs of people and places, handwritten requests, and names of individuals that you want to include in your absentia sendings. These items can be tacked up on a bulletin board or placed inside a wicker basket, healing box, or family photo album.

CHAPTER 9

REIKI SHARES

Part of the healing process is
sharing with other people who care.

Jerry Cantrell

LIKE-MINDED INDIVIDUALS naturally congregate to discuss ideas and share their common interests, and Reiki practitioners are no different. They, too, share a fondness for flocking together. It is Reiki's magnetizing love that invokes an impassioned sense of community among its members, drawing them together. In this chapter, you'll learn about how to participate in (and create) this type of community. You'll learn how Reiki shares offer Reiki practitioners the opportunity to join healing hands in a sacred space. Their combined healing forces not only comfort personal ills but also assist in easing the suffering of all humankind, which means you'll discover how to do more together than you could on your own. Plus, you'll learn how to run a Reiki share in a fair and equitable way.

Learning to Share

Reiki shares, also known as Reiki circles or Reiki exchanges, are occasions that allow Reiki practitioners to gather together to socialize and participate in group healing treatments. The main purpose for the Reiki share is to give and receive Reiki in a casual atmosphere of friendship, honor, and devotion.

During a Reiki share, the recipient lies down on a massage table while the practitioners gather around her and place their hands upon her, facilitating a massive flow of Reiki energies. Group healings are often very powerful and can produce more far-reaching results than individual healer/client Reiki sessions. Because of the increased flow of many combined hands channeling ki energies, a treatment can be completed in a shortened time period of approximately twenty to twenty-five minutes.

Public Reiki Shares

Everyone is welcome to attend publicly sponsored Reiki shares. These shares are often advertised to draw interest from those members of the general public who know little or nothing about Reiki and who might be curious to learn more.

REIKI REFLECTIONS

Public Reiki shares are often held in rented rooms, so there may be a modest fee charged to help cover the costs of the healing space used. Do your homework before you attend a Reiki share by phoning ahead to find out if there are any fees or other special requirements.

Public Reiki shares are ideal places for the Reiki practitioners who have not had many opportunities to treat people outside of their immediate circle of friends and family. Often practitioners come to the shares because they have just started working with Reiki and want to get more experience and confidence when giving a treatment.

You can often find Reiki share invitations and postings available in your area by doing a search on the Internet. A search engine will quickly provide you with many links to help you find just what you are looking for.

REIKI REFLECTIONS

Locating publicly sponsored Reiki shares that are open to the general public is not always easy. Because these shares are free or modestly priced, they are not always well advertised. Look for announcements posted on bulletin boards at public libraries, natural-food markets, wellness centers, and metaphysical bookstores.

Private Reiki Shares

A private share is an informal gathering of individuals who are attuned to Reiki. These types of shares are generally "invitation only" gatherings and are most often held in a home setting. Such shares offer an opportunity for practitioners to work on each other, learn new techniques, and discuss their experiences in working with Reiki. Because the healers normally know each other on a personal level, private shares are much more relaxed than shares that are open to the public.

Private shares are especially helpful to new initiates, giving them a chance to practice the art of Reiki among seasoned healers. Reiki shares offer a safe haven for you to openly ask questions about giving and receiving Reiki in the company of people who understand what you are talking about.

Hosting a Private Reiki Share

Hosting a Reiki share does not require a lot of work, but like most events, it's best to do some preliminary planning. Impromptu shares can be heartfelt as well, but everyone will appreciate the lightness and untroubled atmosphere of a well-organized share.

Taking the time to prepare for your share will make this special healing event more rewarding for everyone involved.

Choosing a Date and Time

Your first step in arranging a share is deciding the date and time of day to hold your share. Choose a day and time that is most convenient for your own schedule. Your personal comfort level should be your primary concern since those attending the share will take their cues from you. If you appear frazzled, rushed, or uncomfortable in any way, this will influence the overall climate of your share environment.

Shares may be arranged for mornings, afternoons, or evenings; they generally last between two and four hours, unless they are all-day affairs. Here are a few typical share schedules:

- Morning Reiki share: 8:30 A.M.–12:00 P.M.
- Afternoon Reiki share: 1:00 P.M.–3:30 P.M.
- Evening Reiki share: 7:00 P.M.–10:00 P.M.
- All-day Reiki share: 10:00 A.M.–8:00 P.M.

The time involved in a share depends on how many people are in attendance, how many tables are being used, and how many treatments are applied. Optimally, each guest will have her turn as a recipient of a treatment from the group before the share concludes.

Inviting Your Guests

Invite your guests at least one week prior to your share date. Private shares are routinely very informal affairs, so formal invitations are not necessary. Inviting your guests can be as easy as making phone calls or sending out e-mails. Of course, if you would like to make your share a special event, invitations sent through the mail are quite elegant.

Your personal invitations may include any special requests that you feel are necessary for the success of the Reiki share. Hosts routinely request their guests to bring something along with them to the share—pillows, a fluffy bolster, healthy drinks or snacks, and so on. If you are in need of a massage table, you may ask a guest to tote along her portable table to help you out. If you already have a table but are planning on a large attendance, you might need someone to bring a second table. You should arrange to have one massage table available for every six or seven guests.

Prepare the Healing Space

If you are a Reiki Level II practitioner, you may send future-event long-distance energies to your event site one day in advance of the share. Add some loving touches, such as flowers from your garden, to the site as well, in order to make the event feel special. On the day of the share, approximately thirty minutes before your guests are scheduled to arrive, take the time to clear and bless the healing space designated for your share. Here are some suggestions for creating a pleasurable environment for your Reiki share:

- Make certain that the room in which you plan to hold your share is free of dust and clutter. Open the windows to let a welcoming breeze into the room if the weather permits.
- Visualize drawing welcoming Cho Ku Rei symbols over the doorways to the room and on the chairs in the space.
- Decorate and harmonize your healing space with feng shui techniques to accentuate your personal tastes. A water fountain gurgling in the background can be a pleasing acoustic touch.

- Having an assortment of colorful and soft pillows scattered about will make everyone feel cozy and pampered.
- Subtly scented incense or aromatherapy candles lit on side tables will enchant the participants of the share.

REIKI REFLECTIONS

Feng shui (pronounced "fung shway") is the ancient Chinese system of arranging living and work environments to allow the maximum flow of energy through them by furniture rearrangement, changes in hues and lighting, and the use of plants and decorative objects to maximize harmony, happiness, and well-being.

You can also conduct a ritual sage smudging to dispel any negative or stagnant energies that may be lingering about. The burning of herbs for emotional, psychic, and spiritual purification is a common practice among many religious, healing, and spiritual groups. The ritual of smudging can be defined as spiritual housecleaning. In theory, the smoke attaches itself to negative energy, and as the smoke clears, it takes the negative energy with it, releasing it into another dimension where it will be regenerated into positive energy.

Nourishment Planning

It is a good idea to have food and drinks available for everyone to snack on between sessions. Think of simple, healthy food options, and steer away from heavy, sugary, or fatty food choices. Here are a few menu ideas to consider:

- Breakfast share menu—Fill a cloth-lined wicker basket with an assortment of freshly baked bagels. Offer your guests their choice of peanut butter or strawberry jam for spreading. Orange-carrot juice or apple cider as the beverage will complete your breakfast menu.
- Afternoon or evening share menu—For a mid-afternoon or evening share, set out small clay bowls filled with dried cherries, golden raisins, and raw almonds. Brew some chamomile or lemon balm herbal tea for their calming properties.
- All-day share potluck—If you are hosting an all-day session, you may opt to prepare a potluck or buffet-style meal. It's a convenient and festive way to share in everyone's favorite foods. You can ask each of the guests to bring along a dish, but be sure that at least some of the dishes can be left out for most of the day. Fresh or dried fruits, unsalted nuts, bran muffins, low-fat yogurt, fruit juices, green drinks, spring water, and herbal teas are excellent nourishment choices.

Setting the Pace

A share group depends on the host to set the pace and flow of the session and treatments. Giving basic instruction to the group will assure that your share functions smoothly.

In order for each person to have his turn at receiving Reiki, divide the time allotted to your share by the number of guests to approximate how long your treatments can last. For example, if you have eight guests and your share is scheduled for three hours, you could break the time down to approximately twenty minutes per treatment. This allows two to three minutes between sessions for stretching legs and bathroom breaks. Keep faithful to your schedule and monitor the time for individual treatments with a wristwatch, minute timer, or wall clock. Designate the person sitting at the head position of the Reiki table to keep track of the minutes allowed for each treatment in order to keep everyone on schedule.

Give each person an opportunity to opt out of a session. Sitting out of the session following one's own healing treatment is sometimes needed to help sort out any issues that may have surfaced. Being able to break away from the healing space relieves the pressure of feeling like you need to give back immediately. Having those few minutes for simply relaxing, eating some food, and perhaps sipping on a cup of tea will help bring you back to the present, revive your spirit, and integrate your overall healing processes.

Reiki Share Etiquette

Most healers subscribe to a code of common courtesy and ethical behavior. Shares are held in sacred healing spaces, and for this reason it is essential that everyone in attendance demonstrate proper respect. The tone need not be too serious, and it should certainly not be stodgy or rigid. Ideally, the atmosphere of a share is one of friendliness, loving, and cordiality.

Honoring Confidences

Whenever giving Reiki, it is important to honor the healing journey of the recipient. You must keep in confidence everything that's shared during the healing session.

Because of the social and informal setting of a share, it can be difficult to determine what is being said in confidence and what is not. If you have difficulty discerning the difference between a recipient processing deep work and merely sharing an amusing family anecdote, it is better not to repeat any of the discussions outside the confines of the share.

Conversation between the practitioners and the recipient is typical and can make a session feel lighter and easier, but getting caught up in excessive chitchat across the table with other guests while disregarding the recipient's healing process on the table is not appropriate or conducive to a successful healing experience.

Focus on the Recipient

Experiencing Reiki is sacred, and each person participates in it in a different way. As you begin each treatment, attempt to make a heart connection with the recipient, maintaining this connection as your primary focus throughout the allotted session time.

Appreciating Your Host

Honor the host for opening up her home and heart in arranging and holding a space for healing. Respect all rules the host has established for the share. Some hosts feel it is ill-mannered for anyone to come to a share and not reciprocate fully in the giving and taking of energies. If you are not able to attend the share for the entire scheduled time, you should inform your host in advance to receive permission to leave the session early.

Shifting Energies

Don't discount or attribute lesser value to share treatments that are of shorter duration than full-body treatments that typically last an hour or longer. Deep levels of energy work can be accomplished in group healings because of the many hands at work.

You will notice a new and different shift of energy taking place as each person lies down on the table to receive his or her

Reiki session. Also, topics of the group's conversation will likely switch from somber to merry and vice versa at the drop of a hat as emotional breakthroughs take place. Because of the empathic nature of many healers, it is not unusual for one or more of them to exhibit emotions that mirror the recipient's experience, such as feeling tearful or melancholy. Keep a box of tissues handy for blowing noses and drying tears of joy and grief.

Shifting of energies during a Reiki share can be quite dramatic and erratic. Imagine taking a six-year-old child to the circus for the first time. The child will be filled with mixed emotions of excitement, chaos, and bewilderment from viewing the clowns, trapeze artists, the fire-eater, and the lion tamer all in one visit. Participating in a Reiki share can be a similarly overwhelming and exhausting experience. This can happen because of the wide range of emotions that are encountered through the different personalities working on their issues. Emotions energetically shared by everyone can include heartbreak, jubilation, depression, sorrow, sexual tension, rejection, and so on.

REIKI REFLECTIONS

The Alexandria Healing Centre in West London advocates the practice of tower healing, a concentrated healing on a desired area. Healers stack their hands, one hand on top of another, forming a tower that beams focused Reiki energies toward the needy area.

Finding a Balance Between Giving and Receiving

Many people have difficulty accepting help or healing. This is especially true of women, particularly mothers, as they are natural givers who don't always know how to receive. Attending shares and allowing yourself to be a receiver of energies will help you find a balance. After attending a few shares and learning to receive, you'll soon be begging to be the first one on the table.

When the Share Is Over

Experiencing a share can leave you feeling as if you are as sleepy and wobbly as a newborn kitten. Because you have soaked up so many energies in a short period of time, it can take you quite a while to assimilate everything you have absorbed. It is important that you disengage and neutralize yourself. Go home and take a shower or bath to refresh your relaxed body and restore your spirit. Drink extra amounts of water for the next twenty-four hours. Remember that water is a purifier, both externally and internally. Give in to your needs. If you feel like taking a nap, give in to that feeling. If you are hungry, feed your body. Absolutely take it easy for the remainder of the day.

Pairing Up with a Partner

All Reiki sessions are about sharing—after all, any Reiki practice bestows love to others (or, in the case of self-treatments, to yourself). Reiki shares are group affairs that involve sharing massive amounts of ki energy. Reiki shared from one person to another can also cultivate a significant amount of light and warmth.

Having another person with whom to share Reiki on a regular basis can be a beneficial way to bring balance into your Reiki regimen. Too often, healers give, give, and give some more, without slowing down long enough to take care of their own needs. By pairing up with another Reiki practitioner and routinely taking turns giving and receiving, each of you will begin to notice symmetry and tranquility in your practice of Reiki.

REIKI REFLECTIONS

Share communities that gather routinely tend to take advantage of the power of group energy and will sometimes spend a few minutes beaming healing energies to planetary concerns such as weather disturbances (earthquakes, tornadoes, drought, floods, and so on) and human crises (war, hunger, poverty, etc.).

Reiki shares can be wonderful outlets for practitioners who are reclusive or introspective types, allowing them to participate in the social atmosphere and gain the advantages of sharing Reiki energies. On the other hand, for practitioners who are inclined to be characteristically more social, a discipline of solitary meditation may be needed to create balance. It is through the quiet use of Reiki that intuition flourishes.

CHAPTER 10

TREATING ACHES AND PAINS

The natural healing force within each one of us is the greatest force in getting well.

Hippocrates

THE ACHES AND PAINS associated with our afflictions are generally our primary concern when we approach treatment. However, our sufferings are much more complex than the dis-eases that afflict the separate components of our physical bodies. In addition to physical discomforts, we suffer from emotional heartbreak and anguish, endure mental stress and anxiety, and struggle with spiritual and moral issues.

In this chapter, you'll learn how Reiki addresses those disturbances that are ready to be released or transformed into positive energy. You'll find out how to deal with physical problems ranging from indigestion to chronic pain through the use of the healing power of Reiki. You'll also explore how to use Reiki to heal mental and emotional difficulties such as anxiety and phobias.

Treating the PEMS Body

When applying spot treatments for injuries, you touch specific areas with the palms of your hands to facilitate a Reiki healing. Remember that Reiki will naturally flow to wherever it is best suited for each individual. This means that the physical dis-ease may or may not be addressed straight away. Reiki may first treat the recipient's emotional trauma or mental distress before directing its attention to any physical damage. Similarly, Reiki could be blocked from working entirely if the recipient is not accepting of it.

REIKI REFLECTIONS

PEMS is an acronym commonly used when referring to our four bodies: physical body, emotional body, mental body, and spiritual body.

Reiki may not immediately heal pains that could be trying to teach us something. This is true with any therapy or healing modality. Our pains teach us to look at our life choices, learned behaviors, or reactions to environmental stimuli, all of which are aspects of life that could possibly need modification. Under these types of life circumstances, Reiki might at first bring about only a release of mental disturbances or emotional flare-ups. This allows the physical manifestation of the dis-ease to linger for a while longer, providing the recipient of the Reiki energy more time to learn tolerance or some other spiritual lesson. Without judgment or expectation on your part, be willing to accept that Reiki flows wherever it is most appropriate and may not affect all parts of your PEMS body.

- Physical body—Reiki is applied to our aches and pains as a means of repairing present dis-eases that have affected the muscular and fleshy tissues, internal organs, and blood and bone elements of our physical bodies. Reiki also speeds the recovery time after surgical procedures and offers pain relief from chronic ailments.
- Emotional body—Reiki serves as a calming agent, and, through its balancing energy, is always ready and able to help disperse and dissolve feelings associated with emotionally charged situations and relationships. Emotional issues eased by Reiki include feelings of rage, fear, abandonment, rejection, and despair.
- Mental body—Reiki offers mental clarity and focus to the confused, distracted, or distraught. Mental distresses such as memory loss, confusion, anxiety, obsessive thoughts, and mania can be placated with the application of Reiki.
- Spiritual body—Reiki is a vehicle that allows us to connect more deeply with our spiritual being. As this spiritual connection deepens, we ultimately arrive at a better understanding of the immense potential we have to heal ourselves.

Treating Common Injuries and Maladies

Normally, there are two basic rules of thumb when it comes to Reiki treatment:

1. Reiki is an intelligent energy that causes no harm.
2. Placing your hands on the body activates Reiki's healing process.

But in addition to these basic rules, you need to keep a few important precautions and exceptions in mind when treating certain types of injuries. These injuries are frequently referred to as the First-Aid Bs: broken bones, bumps and bruises, burns, bleeding, and bee stings.

Treating Broken Bones

If a broken bone is suspected, then a medical evaluation, first and foremost, is warranted. When treating a broken bone, do not place your hands directly over the break. The concern is that Reiki's swift healing process would be a premature remedy to a twisted, splintered, or misaligned injury. It is okay for you to do Reiki over other parts of the body before the bone-setting has taken place, but wait until after the bone has been properly set before applying Reiki directly over the fracture. An energy modality (such as Reiki) alone can't reverse the injury. Reiki should be considered a complementary therapy alongside other healing modalities, rather than an end-all remedy.

REIKI REFLECTIONS

In theory, it could be argued that Reiki is smart enough to reduce only the pain and swelling, refraining from healing the preset bone regardless of where your hands may be positioned. Make your own informed conclusions with this particular teaching.

Treating Bumps and Bruises

Reiki blocks or diminishes bleeding under the skin upon application. Place your hands directly on your stubbed toes, skinned knees, and other bumped areas until the pain subsides. It is important for Reiki to be applied promptly after injury occurs to block or reduce any bruising.

Treating Burns and Sunburns

In the case of a serious burn, medical attention should be sought immediately. Minor burns can be treated with Reiki. When applying

Reiki to burned skin, don't touch it directly. Instead, allow your hands to hover over the burned area at a comfortable distance. You should avoid touching the skin in order to safeguard against possible infection to the burned area. In addition, Reiki energies often generate beaming rays of hot energy. These penetrating streams of hot energy could bring about additional pain or discomfort to the burn victim.

Remember, Reiki energies and symbols can be placed into anything to assist healing and transformation. In treating sunburns you can put healing Reiki rays into aloe vera gel by either holding the bottle between your hands before applying it to the skin or by beaming energies into the gel as it is being distributed to the wound. To protect your skin from the elements, such as dry air and scorching sun rays, you can place Reiki's Harmony symbol, Sei Hei Ki, into sun-block lotions and moisturizing creams.

Treating Bleeding Injuries

For serious or excessive bleeding, first aid and/or immediate medical attention should be sought. Don't touch areas that are bleeding because you could expose the area to possible infections. Also, touching could possibly transfer blood-borne pathogens, such as HIV, hepatitis B, and hepatitis C, from one person to the other.

Treating open cuts and injuries with Reiki to slow or stop the flow of blood is helpful. Actually, Reiki will likely begin to take effect without any intent on your part as you apply bandage pressure on a bloody wound to manage the blood flow. In treating minor cuts, don't be too concerned about stopping the bleeding immediately, since initial bleeding can help cleanse a cut wound of any fragments of metal, glass, or rust that may have become deposited into the wound by the cutting implement. After the injury has been properly cleaned and bandaged, applying hands-on Reiki spot treatment will help hasten restoration.

Treating Insect Stings

Be alert to the potential of dangerous allergies to stings (whether from a bee, wasp, or other insect), symptoms of which include swelling that goes beyond the site of the sting, hives, difficulty breathing or swallowing, swelling of the face or mouth, rapid pulse, or dizziness. Seek prompt medical attention if any of these symptoms occur.

In applying immediate Reiki spot treatment to relieve yourself of the painful burning sensation from a sting, carefully cup or arch your hands over the sensitive area of the body. Be careful not to touch the stung area directly, since this may result in burying the insect's stinger more deeply into the flesh, making it difficult to extract later and possibly leading to an infection. Remove the stinger with sterile tweezers, either before or following the Reiki treatment.

Heartburn and Indigestion

Our digestive systems don't always tolerate the foods that entice our palates. When we overindulge, we can become victims of heartburn, indigestion, nausea, or stomach cramps. Fortunately, the gentle and calming effect of Reiki's energetic flow may ease internal discomforts such as heartburn and upset stomach.

You can quickly neutralize gastric flare-ups by placing your hands upon the chest or abdominal area. Taking a few deep breaths during application will help Reiki break through internal blockages. A good habit to develop is blessing your meals with Reiki before ingestion in order to stave off potential stomach problems.

Treating Hard-to-Reach Areas

Applying hands-on Reiki to certain areas of our bodies for more than a brief period can make one feel like a pretzel and lead to uncomfortable cramping or stiffness in the process. Doing so would not be a problem if you were a trained gymnast or student of yoga, accustomed to bending, stretching, and folding your body in a variety of positions. But for most people, the discomfort of keeping hands placed on certain areas of our bodies for a prolonged period of time can prove burdensome. How many minutes would you be comfortable bent over while keeping your hands on your feet to treat a bunion?

REIKI REFLECTIONS

In Chinese medicine, the meridian healing system is based on the concept that an insufficient supply of ki (chi) makes a person vulnerable to disease. Restoring the ki is the ultimate goal in restoring overall health and well-being to the individual. Acupuncturists, Chinese herbalists, massage therapists, and Reiki practitioners use their various healing methods to assist clients in repairing dysfunctional areas to restore a natural balance.

Being attuned to Level II of Reiki can come in quite handy. When treating hard-to-reach places, Reiki II practitioners can use absentia (distance) treatments to treat the awkward location. Hemorrhoids can be treated successfully by placing your hands on the backside of your surrogate (see Chapter 8) while intentionally beaming warm vibes and healing energies to be transferred to your sore, swollen tissues.

Anxiety and Phobias

Reiki is a practical remedy for calming our fears and reducing anxiety. Even if you are not ordinarily the anxious type, relying on Reiki as a calming agent is a good idea. With the help of Reiki, you may be able to overcome certain phobias, such as the fear of public speaking, death, flying, hospitals, darkness, water, heights, poverty, thunderstorms, or riding in elevators.

Reiki is available 24/7. No matter what type of situation you are facing when fear grips you, Reiki is at your side to help alleviate overcharged energies by bringing in a lower vibration to create a calmer state of mind.

During the course of a day, you may find yourself confronted with situations that frustrate or upset you. Rather than giving in to feelings of impatience when you are caught in heavy traffic and are in a hurry, try placing your hands on yourself and let Reiki bring you some peace and tranquility. Take advantage of any occasions during your daily routine, whether you're standing in line at the supermarket checkout or sitting in the waiting room before a doctor's appointment, to give yourself a Reiki "booster shot." You'll be pleasantly surprised at how quickly any feelings of impatience or frustration will diminish or become dispelled entirely after you allow Reiki to come to your emotional rescue.

For Chronic Pain Sufferers

Chronic pain sufferers consistently seek out new healing modalities to help them manage their dis-eases and discomforts, and for this reason may choose to give Reiki a try. In treating others with chronic pain, don't tout Reiki as a cure-all but rather emphasize that it functions efficiently when used for pain management. Reiki is not a quick fix for a chronic condition. Reiki should be considered a complementary remedy that can safely be used in conjunction with other therapies to assist in healing processes.

Surgical Procedures

Incorporating the use of Reiki when surgery is in the picture will help the intrusive procedure feel less traumatic. Some people have reported that using Reiki resulted in less pain, minimal blood loss during the surgery, and a shortened recovery period.

Prior to surgery, a series of preoperative Reiki treatments can be given to provide comfort and prepare the body for the trauma of being surgically cut and to support the body's own healing processes that will naturally follow. You can also send future-event long-distance energies prior to the time of the scheduled surgery.

During the operation, you can send absentia Reiki to the surgical patient whether you are nearby or far away.

After the operation, the patient may receive a post-operative Reiki treatment in the recovery room. He should continue to receive post-operative Reiki treatments daily for as long as needed to hasten the recovery period.

Living with Terminal Illness

Fighting a terminal illness takes a lot of energy out of a person. Reiki can help replenish lost energy to help in the battle for a better quality of life.

Treating someone with a dreadful dis-ease such as cancer is an act of love that cannot be measured. Channeling large quantities of Reiki energy can be draining, so team up with a group of healers for a healing session.

If you are the sole healer for someone with a terminal illness, please remember to take care of your own needs first. You will not be doing anyone any favors by wearing yourself out. Rather than giving a full treatment in one sitting that would likely involve one or more hours of constant Reiki flow, break the session into fifteen-minute sequences, allowing yourself five to ten minutes of rest between the shorter sessions.

REIKI REFLECTIONS

Reiki, much like prayer, is a personal exercise that can easily convert negative energy into positive energy. For this reason, Reiki is truly a profound and transformative healing experience that can be used to assist a person's transitional journey from the physical earth to that of the spiritual realm. Reiki has also been recognized for the great comfort it offers to the family members and loved ones of someone who is in her final days or who has already passed on.

PART 4

PUTTING IT ALL TOGETHER

When you discover something that nourishes your soul and brings joy, care enough to make room for it in your life.

Jean Shinoda Bolen

In this part, you'll discover how to put all the elements of Reiki together to create a Reiki-centered lifestyle. You'll learn how to enhance your intuition, get in touch with your guides, learn to trust your feelings, and even channel spirits, if you're so moved. You'll begin to understand the importance of seeing Reiki as a spiritual quest.

Next, you'll focus on making Reiki a part of your everyday life by using it to manage your stress, enhance your mood, and affect past, present, and future events. You'll also explore the importance of keeping a Reiki journal.

Finally, you'll learn how to create a Reiki haven at home and how to use Reiki to help your family and to cope with challenges related to family life.

CHAPTER 11

REIKI AND INTUITION

*The more you trust your intuition, the more empowered
you become, the stronger you become,
and the happier you become.*

Gisele Bündchen

INTUITION PLAYS A MAJOR ROLE in the application of Reiki, even though the spiritual component of this healing art is more apparent to some than to others. In this chapter, you'll discover how to use your intuition to aid in healing with Reiki. During Reiki sessions, most practitioners and recipients notice at least some vibrational shifts of energy. Because the source of Reiki's energies is a universal powerhouse, using this energy opens the participants to experiencing deeper aspects of themselves. You'll learn how to recognize these spiritual experiences as they occur, whether that involves noticing subtle cues or realizing awesome inspirations. You'll also discover how intuition allows you to connect with guides, transmute negative energy, and channel spirits.

Connecting with Your Guides

Holding a belief in spirit guides and such is not a requirement for Reiki. Nothing written in this book is designed to convince anyone to change his beliefs. Reiki works whether you believe in it or not—and whether or not you believe in angels, spirit guides, God, Allah, or any other spiritual being or deity.

However, it is important to note that the majority of people who are drawn to Reiki as a hands-on healing art often do tend to be spiritually oriented or religious in some way. They may believe in spirit guides, angels, God, or other deities.

REIKI REFLECTIONS

Some people speak of connecting with new healing energies after becoming attuned to Reiki or having worked regularly with Reiki. They often attribute these energies to spiritual helpers or Reiki guides.

Communicating with Higher Aspects

Everyone has the ability to communicate with "higher aspects" of himself, with or without using Reiki. Higher aspects represent whatever higher power you are aligned with: God, angels, animal totems, spirit guides, higher self, soul-body, heart center, inner dialogue, and so on.

The attunement process that takes place in Reiki classes clears away blockages in the physical body, helping these loftier types of communications to occur more easily. Through continued use of Reiki, the passageways in your body through which the ki energies flow broaden, creating a direct communication avenue, similar to a pipeline or telegraph wire, with the Reiki guides.

Reiki guides provide practitioners with the information needed to assist them in applying Reiki treatments. As the Reiki practitioner further develops his intuitive abilities, the Reiki guides orchestrate the healing sessions more and more in order to allow the healing energies to operate with greater fluidity. They direct where the Reiki practitioner's hands need to be placed on the recipient's body and when the hand placements should be changed. Finally, they suggest what kinds of questions to ask the recipient to further assist the practitioner in conducting a proper and thorough Reiki treatment. It is through this guidance that a practitioner is able to connect with the "soul-body" of his recipient and more fully support the recipient in her healing journey.

REIKI REFLECTIONS

You may not "see" your angels or spirit guides. Not everyone acquires spiritual guidance visually. Pay attention to extrasensory spiritual messages. When we neglect to notice the simpler messages conveyed by a spirit that needs our attention, these communications will eventually be demonstrated in more recognizable ways that you may not appreciate.

False Expectations of Reiki Guides

Some Reiki II classes are promoted with the assurance that the students will meet their Reiki guides as a part of the class curriculum. Some teachers even lead guided meditations, inviting the Reiki guides to join their class sessions. As a result, some students sign up for Reiki classes not so much to learn the healing art but to miraculously be connected with their guides. Naturally, those students who are not able to instantly "see" or "hear" their guides become disappointed. Frustrations are compounded when other Reiki initiates share personal stories of their own guide connections during the class sessions. The students who do not forge a connection with their Reiki guides assume that there is something wrong with them or that the Reiki attunement didn't work. This is not the case. It is best not to make assumptions about what will or won't happen on your Reiki journey.

REIKI REFLECTIONS

Our expectations in life are often what trip us up. This is especially true when you pair expectations with Reiki. It is best to approach Reiki with no expectations and allow your personal experience with it to unfold naturally.

Listening to Your Inner Dialogue

Each of us is unique in how we intuit information. Learning to tune in to your inner dialogue takes some practice. Allow your expectations to melt away. Figuratively speaking, lean your ear against your heart and listen intently. Here are a few suggestions for flexing your intuition muscles:

- Expand your intuitive ear by quieting your physical ears. Turn off your radio, stereo, and television. Spend a half-hour each day in quiet meditation or solitude.
- Go for nature walks by yourself. Allow your psyche to merge with sounds of the forest, seashore, mountain trail, and other natural wonders.
- Pay attention to energy shifts in your physical body. Pain is a signifier that something is wrong.
- Keep a dream journal. Dreams are one of the easiest avenues through which intuitive messages are filtered.

- Take a moment every day to clear away unproductive thoughts and to release cerebral distractions and obsessive mental chatter. Visualize a chalkboard being erased of these thoughts.
- Keep a synchronicity diary to write down all the "coincidences" you experience throughout the day.
- Follow your hunches. Prepare to be amazed where they lead you.
- Pay attention to what emotions or memories are invoked when you are around specific scents.
- Start noticing markers or signs that bring about particular sensations in your gut.

However, don't get overly preoccupied with figuring out the reasons for every little thing that happens in your daily life. Don't worry if you begin to perceive messages that you don't fully understand right away. Explanations tend to come along with intuitive messages on a "need to know" basis. Using your sixth sense is just like flexing a muscle. It will get stronger the more you exercise it.

Emotional Centers of the Body

The strongest "feeling centers" in the body are the heart and the solar plexus region. The heart is the place from which our love of self and love for others flow. This is also the area where our emotional hurts and wounds are stored.

In Touch with Your Heart

There is no right or wrong feeling that comes from the heart. These feelings are what they are, pure and simple. No shame or blame should be placed upon anyone because of the way she feels— whether it's love or hate, humility or anger, happiness or sadness, guilt or grief, calm or fear and anxiety. Acknowledging one's feelings without judgment is the first step toward healing heart wounds.

Learning forgiveness, trust, unconditional love, and compassion are spiritual challenges associated with the heart region. Emotional empowerment can be achieved by releasing repressed negative feelings that shadow our purest and most positive emotions.

A Heart-to-Heart Exercise

A heart-to-heart communication can be intuited while giving a Reiki treatment. The following exercise can be an overwhelming emotional experience for the practitioner because of the outpouring of love that is transferred from the recipient's heart into the practitioner's. The outcome can be quite profound.

While applying the throat and heart hand placements on the recipient's body, focus on your own heart. Visualize your heart chakra spinning in a clockwise motion. While it continues to spin, shift your focus to the recipient's heart and visualize her heart chakra spinning in a clockwise motion as well. Imagine both heart chakras spinning in unison and connecting with one another.

Open your heart and listen for any messages that are intuitively conveyed. Pay close attention to the messages as if you are a parent listening to your beloved son or daughter, keeping any information received strictly confidential. Silently acknowledge that you totally accept the recipient just as she is. From your heart, extend your unconditional love to the recipient.

On a Hunch

Your inner knowledge originates in the solar plexus. This region of the body defines your self-esteem and personal power. Strong self-esteem is a requirement for developing intuitive skills. When you choose to ignore your gut instincts, you are only hurting yourself further by distrusting messages that are meant to help you. The more often you allow yourself to follow the direction of your gut feelings, the clearer the intuitive pathway will become. By following through on everyday hunches, no matter how unimportant they may seem, you are actually taking test drives, virtually honing your intuitive listening skills.

Trusting Your Feelings

Information from a spiritual source often comes through as if the message is written in a foreign language or secret code, and yet you must try to read and comprehend it. Not only that, but there is no translator present to help you crack the code or understand the message.

Interpreting these confusing messages can be challenging. Generally, the analytical brain wants to jump in and decipher the messages using methodical reasoning, but this often creates more confusion.

To interpret intuitive messages, you need to process them with your emotional body rather than with your mental faculties. What feeling did the message invoke in you? Sadness? Happiness? Loneliness? Confusion? Did it bring up repressed feelings from an unresolved issue? Once you can identify the feeling, you will have something to work with.

Emotional Release

A Reiki treatment is often the trigger that elicits messages to help a person get in touch with the feelings that need to be expressed. By invoking the Hon Sha Ze Sho Nen, or Connection, symbol, you can direct Reiki to delve deeper into any feelings that have surfaced from within the recipient.

Occasionally a person will experience an intense emotional release during or after a Reiki treatment. These types of emotional releases may be expressed through crying, screaming, coughing, or even laughing. Emotional releases help carry the person through the hurts and discomforts associated with the feelings that arise during a Reiki session.

Sharing Communication

When you intuit messages from your Reiki guides concerning the recipient you're treating, it is up to you to decide whether or not to pass on these messages to the recipient. Trust your feelings in making these decisions. Sometimes the guides provide the practitioner with particular information during a treatment in order to assist him in the healing itself. At other times, the guides intend the messages to be shared with the recipient.

Sometimes the information that comes through will not make sense to you. If it has a feeling of urgency or persistence attached to it, the message probably needs to be shared with the recipient. Although the message might not make sense to you, it might have a special meaning to the recipient. Sometimes the recipient is not open to receiving intuited information directly, and the practitioner will serve as a channel through which a recipient's spirit guides can pass on communications.

Are You an Empath?

Natural empaths are individuals who feel the emotions and physical ailments of the people around them. As children, empaths are often called "overly sensitive" because their feelings are easily hurt and they have difficulty controlling their emotions. As a result, many learn to shield themselves from absorbing other people's emotions. As empathic children become adults, they may have difficulty lowering their protective walls in order to form loving relationships.

REIKI REFLECTIONS

Traits of a natural empath include sensitivity, compassion, good listening skills, a need to serve as a peacemaker to others, a strong sense of caution, and a quiet, guarded disposition.

Empathy As a Healing Tool

You may acquire and develop an empathic awareness as you practice Reiki. Empathic Reiki practitioners use the intuited information to assist them in their hand placements and in directing the flow of Reiki. However, you need to be able to discern the difference between feeling the recipient's ailments and experiencing your own health issues. If you feel general discomfort during a treatment, ask the recipient how she feels. For example, if you get a cramp in your leg or suddenly feel nauseated, ask the recipient if she is experiencing the discomfort as well. After you realize that a pain or discomfort you are experiencing doesn't belong to you, release it as quickly as possible. Do not continue to hold on to it.

REIKI REFLECTIONS

Although empaths "feel" others' pain, they do not actually take it away from others. An empath merely intuits information with regard to how the other person is feeling. In shamanic healing methods, the shaman will take the client's issues and physical problems into his body for transmutation and transformation. This specialized healing technique should not be used without extensive training.

Releasing Empathized Illnesses

Feeling the recipient's illness in this way can be invaluable in understanding her state of health. However, you must not hold those energies in your body any longer than necessary. Acknowledge the empathized information that was offered, silently thank your spirit source for the knowledge its guidance has offered you, and ask that the discomfort be released from your body.

Allow the discomfort to fade away as you continue treating the recipient. If the empathized feeling does not subside and your discomfort continues, you may need to disconnect from the recipient for a few seconds by removing your hands from her body. In severe cases, you may need to discontinue the treatment altogether.

You may feel conflicted between wanting to intuit feelings to help treat someone and not wanting to feel the discomfort. In that case, you should shield yourself entirely from taking on illnesses. The Reiki Harmony symbol, Sei Hei Ki, is a protection symbol used to help create walls between you and the people you treat. Allowing yourself to take on others' illnesses is putting yourself at risk until you have either learned how to shield yourself or have become accomplished at quickly releasing these ills and discomforts.

Transmuting Negative Energies

Reiki treatments often cause emotional and mental issues that might have become trapped or buried in the recipient's body to surface. This offers an opportunity for any negative and stagnant energies to move upward and outward. However, these energies should be transmuted and transformed into positive energy before they are allowed to re-enter the universe, where they might inadvertently affect someone else. If you have ever walked into an empty room and felt a negative emotional charge (we may call these negative charges "bad vibes"), you have experienced what it is like to suddenly come upon discharged energy that has not been transmuted. Leaving discharged negative energy out in the open for others to stumble over is equivalent to leaving smelly garbage out on your street or dumping your dirty laundry for others to trip over.

During the treatment, anytime you feel discharged energy accumulating, take a moment to energetically clear the auric field. Always conclude a full-body treatment this way. And clear your healing space between Reiki treatments as well.

To clear the auric field, comb the recipient's aura to clear it of any energy debris that has lifted from the physical body during the treatment. To do this, move your hands in multiple circular motions or in feathering sweeps over the recipient's body. As you sweep away the debris, you may want to make a prayerful request for the negative energies to be transmuted and transformed into positive energies to be used for universal goodness. Some healers will send these energies to the "white light" to be purified and transformed.

REIKI REFLECTIONS

White light is the space within the universe that is filled with positive energies. White light can be used only for good purposes and can be called upon for protection from negative energies. It can neither come to harm nor cause harm. When anything is sent to the white light, it is balanced and charged with positive energy.

Channeling Spirits

Receiving any type of spiritual communication is a form of channeling. However, the term "channeling" normally means that a person is being used as a human loudspeaker to communicate information from a particular spirit to one or more people and sometimes to the world at large.

There are two types of spirit channeling—trance channeling and conscious channeling. Trance channelers are able to set aside their conscious selves in order to loan their bodies for communication with another energy form. These energy forms have many names: spirit guides, spirit entities, Ascended Masters, and so on. Conscious channelers do not give up their conscious selves entirely when they allow information to be channeled through them. Communications that are the result of conscious channeling will have a certain percentage of distortion because it is censored to some degree by the channeler's personality.

During the Reiki attunement process, the avenue within the body that is opened to allow Reiki to flow through also opens up the psychic communication centers. This is why many Reiki practitioners report having channeled communications with the spirit world. In some cases, practitioners claim to have received additional information regarding the Reiki system through their channeling.

A Spiritual Quest

Many a spiritual seeker has stumbled across Reiki while making the journey through life. Reiki, along with its principles, is quickly accepted as a valuable find that assists anyone who wants to continue along the pathway toward well-being and self-discovery. Many people, after immersing themselves in the teachings of Reiki, adopt Reiki as their ultimate way of life.

CHAPTER 12

INTEGRATING REIKI INTO EVERYDAY LIFE

Every religion emphasizes human improvement, love, respect for others, sharing other people's suffering. On these lines every religion has more or less the same viewpoint and the same goal.

Dalai Lama

AS A REIKI PRACTITIONER who embraces all of Reiki's principles and conducts healings on a regular basis, you will most likely enjoy a more fulfilling life than you would otherwise. In this chapter, you'll learn how Reiki can be integrated into all aspects of your daily life to assist you in meeting your goals and to help you deal with any problems that arise. The purpose of this chapter is to help you understand how to create a Reiki-centered life, which is more than just giving and receiving Reiki treatments. Here, you'll learn how to call upon Reiki's stress-reducing energies whenever you are confronted with episodes of anxiety, adversity, or affliction in your everyday life. You'll also learn how to use Reiki energy to heal past hurts, stay present, and help ensure positive outcomes for future events.

A Part of Your Every Day

A common question students ask in a Reiki class is, "How can I squeeze a daily full-body Reiki treatment into my already hectic twenty-four-hour day?" They can't see how Reiki will fit into their world without upsetting their established routines. The answer: adjustment and integration.

Inviting Reiki into your life is much like welcoming a new baby into your family. At first, the introduction of Reiki energies within your body will likely upset your routines. You may find yourself losing sleep or you may discover that you need more sleep than normal.

Reiki treats imbalances in the body to bring about overall good health and well-being. If your body lacks sleep, diet, exercise, or something else, Reiki energies will accordingly cause drowsiness, stimulate food cravings, or promote the desire to take a walk or start lifting weights. These changes begin at the onset of the Reiki attunement process. For some people, routines will change drastically; for others, only slight changes occur. How dramatic or subtle the changes will be depends on the degree of balancing needed to create level and calm energies.

As you continue to practice Reiki, your routines will shift as needed and eventually stabilize to a new normal that is appropriate for you. Your body will learn to adjust to and welcome the relief Reiki offers in aligning your energies on a regular basis. Whenever you feel sick or tense, rather than telling yourself to relax or reaching for that bottle of pain-relief pills, simply place your hands on your body to allow calm and peace to equalize your upsets.

Using Reiki to Manage Your Stresses

Reiki, when used routinely, can help manage your stresses. It helps because Reiki's balancing energies will promptly address those blips on the emotional flux radar screen as soon as they appear.

Life isn't always easy. No one glides through life without experiencing some difficult times. Deal with occasional stressful situations by remaining open to the flow of Reiki. Keeping your body free of energy blocks will help you deal with and process stresses more efficiently whenever they arise.

It is natural for you to want to invite Reiki into your life and to treat yourself when sick or feeling troubled. However, Reiki isn't a salve in a tube that sits in a first-aid kit until an accident or emergency occurs. Reiki should be applied daily to supplement your well-being much like a multivitamin supplements your dietary health. Reiki, applied routinely, can help keep life-stimulating energies from getting bogged down or becoming completely stagnant within your body.

Because Reiki's ki energies are inherently always in motion, it only makes sense that a person who routinely invites Reiki to flow freely through her body is going to feel less threatened when an obstacle pops up in the course of what, at first, seems to be a perfect day.

Anyone whose nature normally resists "going with the flow" can become more "flowing" with the assistance of Reiki.

Unexpected occurrences in your daily life can bring about feelings of anxiety or uncertainty. Going with the flow is the easiest pathway to avoid stresses. Your anxiety-ridden reaction may be to jump off the train before the train derails. But wait! You boarded this train to experience the journey, so don't panic. You'll survive this; just let the dust settle first. Then, allow Reiki to help pull you through.

Whenever you feel yourself losing control with the possibility of reacting with little or no forethought, sit tight. Place the palms of your hands on your heart and solar plexus, take one or two deep breaths, and allow Reiki to calm you.

With Reiki at your side, you can keep a cool head during a crisis. It's not that you won't feel stress—you probably will. But you'll be able to draw on Reiki's infinite flow of healing energies to keep you level-headed with a steady heartbeat and balanced demeanor. Reiki can, and absolutely will, help you maintain a healthy balance in the most stressful conditions when you apply it with care and confidence.

Mood Enhancement and Meditation

Mind-body connection studies have proved that a regular course of meditation improves the function of the immune system as well as offering other medical benefits. Meditation techniques may include any of the following:

- Vocalizing repetitive mantras
- Focused awareness and/or control of the breath

- Listening to music
- Practicing imagery and visualization
- Participating in active meditative-style exercises such as dance, kundalini yoga, and tai chi

Reiki energies complement all meditative approaches that people use to promote well-being.

Reiki Visualization Vacation

Whether you need to quash depressive thoughts or calm over-stimulated nerves, imaginative visualization may be the solution. If you find it easy to mentally visualize the Reiki symbols, you will enjoy playing with these symbols during your meditations. Imagery play can be a welcome escape from the mundane or frustrating events and toils of daily life. Taking a ten-minute visual vacation away from your stressful life can certainly revive depressive moods.

Allow the Reiki Connection symbol, Hon Sha Ze Sho Nen, to be the magic carpet that carries you off to faraway places. Focus on a desired destination, draw the symbol, and mentally send the energy to that place, with yourself tagging along for the ride.

Another imaginative visualization you can try is to imagine a large Hula-Hoop floating horizontally in the air above you. The hoop represents a vortex opening into a different reality. Visualize the Power symbol, Cho Ku Rei, floating inside the circular hoop. Next, imagine yourself jumping up into the hoop and through the Power symbol into a new reality of your making. This reality can be a revisit to your childhood, a swim date with a school of dolphins, or an explorative tour through an enchanted castle. With the help of this visualization, you can go virtually anywhere your mind will take you.

Pumping Ki

Breath awareness exercises and physical workouts are two excellent activities that will help open up your ki passages prior to giving or receiving a Reiki treatment. Choose exercises that remind you of play—most people tend to prefer activities that are joyous and fun to those that feel laborious or bothersome.

A favorite ki breath exercise is to sit upright with your spine straight, open your mouth, relax your jaw, stick out your tongue, and pant like a dog. The in-and-out breaths will open up your belly and clear the ki passageways from the base of your spine to your throat's vocal cords.

An enjoyable physical exercise that will free up knots and kinks in the spine is to rock your body back and forth like a rocking chair. Position your body comfortably on a yoga mat or carpeted floor. Bend your knees and bring them close to your chest. Wrap your arms around your knees and begin rocking your body back and forth. This movement massages your back's bones and muscles. It also effectively opens up the ki channels that run along your spine. Best of all, it's easy and simply fun to do, almost like being a kid again.

Book a Reiki Session

Doing self-treatments is a wonderful way to value yourself and to honor your body, but sometimes we crave touch and caring from another individual in order to feel fully loved and pampered. Swapping treatments with other practitioners is one option. If you are traveling or visiting a new town, try to locate a Reiki practitioner in the area and treat yourself to a full-body treatment. You may discover a new friend as well as learn a new healing technique in the process. It will also make your stay in a strange place more pleasurable.

Past, Present, and Future Events

At various times throughout any given day, our thoughts tend to drift back and forth from our past experiences to our future planned events. While we are mentally revisiting childhood memories or needlessly fretting about next week's deadline at work, we overlook the here and now of our life today.

Reiki has access to both your past and your future. It will flow beyond present-day ailments, delving deeply into the body to heal past hurts. And Reiki's distance formula can also be used to offer positive energies to future events.

In the Past

It is our past experiences that have helped form our personalities. Who we are today, or, put another way, what we have made of ourselves, is the result of the culmination of all our past experiences. Reiki can be directed at specific memories to heal energies surrounding those experiences that negatively influence the current personality.

The Reiki Connection symbol, Hon Sha Ze Sho Nen, gives the adept Reiki practitioner the tool to access the Akashic Records. Here the practitioner can obtain information on hurts and ills that are lingering in the body from past experiences. These lingering hurts may date back to last week, last month, last year, or much farther back in time—as far back as your childhood and past-life experiences.

For example, Reiki can be directed to treat the lingering fear of a person who had a traumatic first day at school. This is an example of inner-child therapy. You can use a teddy bear surrogate to facilitate your own inner-child work. Rather than doing a full-body treatment, sit quietly with a stuffed teddy bear on your lap or hold a hand-sized bear between the palms of your hands. Use the distance formula and send Reiki to the small child within you who needs love, understanding, and healing. Spend at least an hour on this to fully give your inner child the care so desperately craved.

In the Future

You can also send Reiki ahead to smooth the way for you before embarking on a particular venture or journeying to a specific place. Here are a few examples of future events that you may wish to energize using a Reiki distance treatment:

* Academic exams
* Blind dates
* Family gatherings

- Giving birth
- Job interviews
- Medical appointments
- School reunions
- Speaking engagements
- Sports tournaments
- Talent shows

You won't feel as lonely, fearful, or lost if confronted with new experiences when you have Reiki energies awaiting you to make your transition into a strange or uncomfortable situation easier. The Reiki warms up the space and helps your communications with others as future events unfold.

Journal Your Reiki Experiences

For centuries, people have been relying on diaries, travelogues, and scrapbooks to document their histories, pilgrimages, experiences, and individual insights. Recording your Reiki experiences by writing them down in a notebook or private journal is a good way to track energy shifts and personal growth changes that occur. Your Reiki journal need not be anything fancy, nor need your scribblings be profound. Simply jot down notes in a handy pocket notebook, keep a private diary, or publish an online blog.

Dedicating Your Journal

For every adventure embarked upon, there is both anticipation and apprehension surrounding it. You may experience ambiguous emotions because you're not sure how and why events and experiences will eventually unfold. Being newly attuned to Reiki is very much like starting a new page or new chapter in your life. Why not grab an empty notebook and keep a log of this new adventure as it plays out? If you've been practicing Reiki for a while, it's never too late to pick up the habit of keeping a journal. Even if you have not yet begun to document your Reiki journey, there is no better time than now.

When you begin your journal, dedicate it to someone or some purpose. Here are a few sample suggestions:

- "I dedicate this book to my Reiki guides and to the inner child within me who wants to get out and play more often."
- "I dedicate this book to my Reiki Master and my own journey following her wise and wandering footsteps."
- "This Reiki journal is dedicated to the creativity that stirs within me. May I always pursue joy."

REIKI REFLECTIONS

You are a work in process; in other words, you are growing with Reiki. The journal will serve as a yardstick that measures how far you've come, and it will continue to grow with you.

Three Steps to Starting Your Reiki Journal

After selecting a notebook, binder, or journal book to use for your Reiki writings, you might find yourself staring down at the blank pages and wondering how to begin filling in the pages. Or, perhaps your creative juices are overflowing and you are itching to get started putting pen to paper. Either way, begin your journal experience by first putting your unique stamp on it; second, by writing out the history of your personal Reiki beginnings; and third, by making an intention statement.

Put Your Unique Stamp on It

Put your own unique identifying mark on your journal. Fill the first couple of pages with information about yourself and what your reasons are for bringing Reiki into your life. Paste a photograph of yourself on the cover or on the inside cover of the journal. This journal is about Reiki, but more so, its purpose is to track your Reiki pilgrimage. The primary focus of keeping a Reiki journal is you and your personal experiences and sentiments when using Reiki. You and Reiki are the two staple ingredients in this endeavor, with you serving as the storyteller. It is important that you recognize your own value in this process.

Write about Your Reiki Beginnings

After you personalize your journal, the second step is for you to write down your reasons for taking a Reiki class and what your initial expectations are for choosing Reiki. Write down your impressions of your teacher. What types of emotions were you feeling during the class? Describe your reactions to the attunement process. Did you sense a rapport with any of your classmates, or did you sense agitation with some classmates?

Continue to write, write, and write some more. Don't worry if you are rambling or wandering off subject. You are not writing a manuscript that is going to be published. This journal-keeping exercise is meant for your own personal use. Think of it as a private forum where you can express your feelings freely. No one is going to grade it or reprove you for messy handwriting.

Make Your Intention Statement

The third step is to write out an intention statement. State your intention clearly and concisely. Here are a few sample intention statements, although you should certainly feel free to create your own:

- "It is my intent to use Reiki in my life in order to develop a deeper relationship with my personal awareness."
- "I choose to embrace Reiki with all that I am."
- "It is my intent to create a healthier, wealthier, and happier life for my family and me."

Bless Your Journal

Next, bless your Reiki journal by holding it between both of your hands and allowing Reiki energies to flow freely from your palms into its pages. If you've been attuned to Level II Reiki, you may also add Reiki symbols in your journal. Keep your book in a handy place, such as inside your desk drawer or on top of your bedside table, where you can readily find it and add entries to it on a regular basis.

Letting Creativity Flow

You have completed steps one, two, and three. Now the instruction ends. There are no steps numbered four, five, and six. The continuation of this journal project is entirely up to you. Actually, you can ignore steps one, two, and three, if you like, and create your own steps to begin with. Those initial three steps are only meant as a framework to get you started.

The true treasure within creative journal writing is that there are no steadfast rules. A poet will fill his journal with impromptu prose and beautiful poetry. The artist's journal pages will be adorned with drawings and sketches. The neat person will likely keep her journal tidy and well organized, with little fluff or doodle clutter. The free-spirited individual will sprinkle his notebook with frills and spontaneous journal entries. Your goals should be to express your emotions and to document your Reiki experiences.

REIKI REFLECTIONS

Your journal doesn't have to be filled with pages and pages of text. You can add drawings, pictures, doodles, and diagrams if that will help you better express yourself. Keep a set of markers or colored pencils next to your journal, and use them to enhance your written entries whenever the mood strikes you.

Personal Growth

It can be remarkably interesting to turn back to your first journal entries a few weeks, months, or perhaps years after they were written and review your recorded thoughts and feelings about your Reiki experiences. Sometimes we are impatient, feeling as if we are spinning our wheels in this life. We want changes to occur instantly. Going back in time and reading your early journal entries will help you better understand that life has not stood still. The concerns and troubles that were bothering you early on will likely not seem so important or overwhelming to you later. In fact, many of those ruts in the road and tricky stumbling blocks will have faded away completely. You will discover that your goals and initiatives will have been met or ultimately changed into something entirely different. Our priorities change as life advances. Reiki can help put all of our priorities in order.

Documenting Reiki Sessions

Track your Reiki self-treatments by recording or documenting them. By reviewing your notes, you will get concrete clues as to what healing techniques work best for you. You may also learn what time of the day is more favorable for conducting treatments, better understand what kinds of results can be realized, and begin to carve out basic groundwork that will benefit future treatments.

Treatment notations can be blended into your other journal entries. Label or highlight them in some way so that they can easily be identified as you thumb through your journal pages. If you are using a three-ring binder, you may find it helpful to keep a separate divider section for your self-treatment notes.

Dreams and Manifestations

Think of your journal as the perfect garden spot wherein you lovingly nurture and elegantly cultivate your expressed dreams and desires. Reiki is one of the grandest manifestation tools available today and can be very powerful. Reiki manifestations will even work for those "seeing is believing" types if they are willing to give it a try. All you need to do is follow these simple steps:

1. Dream it.
2. Write it down.
3. Stamp your intention on it.
4. Focus on it.
5. Apply Reiki to it.
6. It manifests!

Naturally, Reiki manifestations can be limited or blocked, but they are only limited or blocked because of the limits or barriers that we impose on them. Those limitations and barriers are of our own making and never originate within Reiki itself.

CHAPTER 13

CREATING A REIKI HAVEN AT HOME

*Every day is a journey,
and the journey itself is home.*

Matsuo Basho

THE WORLD WOULD BE A CALMER and friendlier place if all family members were attuned to Reiki and practiced it regularly. In this chapter, you'll learn how both residence and relationships benefit greatly from love energies freely flowing from room to room and person to person. You'll find out why you should go ahead and put out the welcome mat and invite Reiki into your life as a cherished member of the family. If you do, you'll begin to notice less tension, fewer arguments, and more laughter when Reiki is allowed to work its magic. You'll also find helpful advice for dealing with common problems and challenges in families. In other words, you'll discover everything you need to know to make your home a Reiki-centered space. This chapter focuses on practicing Reiki with other family members who also share your interest in energy healing and on how to incorporate it into your home. Reiki thrives anywhere it is welcome, making its energies easily accessible.

Home Sweet Home

Create the intention to make your own home a Reiki haven. Basically, you can infuse your home with Reiki healing energies by touching everything in sight. Reiki your house plants, family pets, furniture, and appliances. Reiki the entryways, stairwells, closets, and pantries. Reiki the bed pillows and mattresses. The list of tangibles that you can infuse with the energy of Reiki within your home is endless.

In order to truly make Reiki a way of life, use Reiki to treat all the environments in which you spend your time. Whether you are at home, work, the grocery market, health clinic, or anywhere else, you can increase the comfort level for yourself and everyone else in that environment simply by inviting Reiki to dwell there with you.

Before walking into any sort of building, visualize a large Reiki Power symbol drawn in the building's entrance doorway. As you enter the building, you will walk through this freshly drawn Power symbol. Walking through eight-foot-tall Cho Ku Rei symbols can feel extremely empowering.

REIKI REFLECTIONS

When traveling, you can incorporate the use of Reiki's Protection symbol as a cautionary measure to help safeguard your luggage and its contents from loss or damage.

Giving Reiki to any designated space is an interesting experiment for you to try. Results will vary depending on the current energy state of the particular space you select and on the occupants of that space. Optionally, you can send Reiki in advance to any place you plan to visit later by visualizing the symbols and directing a distance treatment.

Reiki and Your Sex Life

Our physical bodies allow us, as spiritual beings, to experience human existence. Why would we strive to shed our physical garb and lose the opportunity to have this unique experience? Celibacy is a choice that can help a person develop his personal awareness. Some Reiki practitioners choose celibacy, while others are sexually active.

The sacral chakra (located just below the tailbone) determines our sexual appetites and disposition. It is also associated with our playfulness and our creative natures. Spiritual lessons associated with the sacral chakra are creativity, manifestation, honoring relationships, and learning to let go.

The attunement process that activates Reiki moves the ki energies through all the chakras. The energy movement begins at the crown chakra and moves downward through the root chakra and back up again. Any chakras that are shut down or partially blocked will be opened up during the attunement. The sacral chakra, the body's sexual center, cannot help but be affected by this. This is especially true if it had not been functioning fully beforehand. If a person has been sexually repressed or has had his sexual center shut down, the Reiki attunement could very possibly open up a Pandora's box of intimacy-related issues, sexual urges, and emotions.

A person can have an active sex life even when his sacral chakra is blocked or shut down. Basically, a person with a closed sexual center goes through the motion of having sex without having a total awareness of his body. Having sex in this way can be enjoyable, but it does not compare to having a sexual experience with the sacral chakra open. Sharing sexual intimacy while your sacral chakra is open and functioning can be a completely startling experience for someone who has been closed off from his physical body.

Turning Your Partner On with Reiki

Reiki and sexual intimacy go together beautifully. The Reiki practitioner who conducts regular self-treatments will keep his chakras in perfect working order. When your sacral chakra is open and functioning, it can work like an attraction beacon that will bring you and your lover together like a pair of magnets. Your lover may not realize why she is being drawn so strongly to you; she will just know that being around you makes her feel good.

Bringing Reiki energy into your lovemaking is not only a wonderful gift for yourself but will also be appreciated by your partner. If you and your partner are both attuned to Reiki, your lovemaking has the potential to blend your energies together in sacred sexuality; in other words, it will be a union of two souls.

Reiki Body Massage

Giving your partner a Reiki massage is an open-hearted and nurturing demonstration of your love. For some couples, it may be a good way to arouse each other sexually. For others, it may have a calming, relaxing effect, easing the stresses from the recipient's body and sending them right into a slumber pose. Whether you use it for foreplay or before sleep, Reiki massage is a wonderful way to be intimate with your partner.

The basic Reiki hand placements are not used while giving a massage. Reiki will naturally kick in during the session. For instance, you can lovingly give your partner a Reiki back rub:

1. Charge your (preferably organic) massage oils with Reiki energies. Sweet almond oil and jojoba oil are favorites for releasing stresses.
2. Have your partner lie on her stomach on a bed.
3. Cover the lower part of your partner's body with some warm towels or a light blanket so she will not be chilled.
4. Pour a handful of massage oil in your hands. Allow your Reiki hands to warm the oil.
5. Begin by smoothing your hands in slow, sweeping movements across your partner's neck, shoulders, and upper back.
6. Begin stroking and rubbing the neck and shoulders.
7. Continue kneading out any kinks or stresses as you move your hands down your partner's back.
8. Finish the massage by lightly scratching her skin surface with your fingernails in circular or figure-eight movements.
9. Lie down and snuggle up next to your partner.

The back rub massage described here should not be used as therapy in a clinical setting or as a healing practice. Such behavior is not acceptable between a practitioner and a client and should be reserved for your intimate relationship.

Help for Couples Experiencing Infertility

When a couple is coping with infertility, the repeated cycles of disappointment can be emotionally wearing and adversely affect overall well-being. This is where Reiki can come to the rescue. Routine Reiki treatments will help balance the roller coaster of emotions associated with fertility problems for both men and women. It can also be used to complement a variety of other alternative treatments that promote fertility, such as massage or acupuncture. Reiki can also assist in balancing hormonal ups and downs that coincide with in vitro fertilization (IVF) treatments.

Tool for Weathering Emotional Storms

Reiki is not a cure for infertility or anything else for that matter. The words "cure" and "miracle" are sometimes spoken in regard to Reiki, but it is best to keep these terms in check. Using Reiki routinely can open up a space for a healing, a cure, or even a miracle. You may read or hear about couples who credit Reiki for their thrust into parenthood, but the science to prove this just isn't available to confirm it. The last thing that couples experiencing infertility need to hear are promises that cannot be kept.

Not every couple challenged with infertility who tries Reiki will be blessed with a bundle of joy for their efforts. However, Reiki is a useful tool for helping to weather any emotional storms you are caught up in. Emotions connected with infertility can go on for months or even years. It dumps energetic debris in its path. Couples experiencing infertility will often feel pushed to the very limits of their endurance and patience.

Relationships can become fragile under all the stress and emotional upheaval of trying to conceive. Baby-making sex is not as relaxing or enthralling as sex for the sake of pleasure and intimacy. Emotions associated with infertility can certainly have a negative effect on one's sex life. Again, Reiki may or may not be your ticket into parenthood, but it can definitely be of service by soothing downtrodden spirits and calming spiked anxieties associated with couples who are struggling with infertility.

Nurture Your Nurturing Needs

A couple can get so caught up in trying to have a baby that they will have forgotten the reason why they wanted to become parents in the first place. Or perhaps they never were clear about why. You can know you want to be a parent without really understanding why. A primary reason for wanting to be a parent or to practice parenthood is to have someone in their lives to care for and nurture.

You will not be emotionally prepared to welcome a baby into your arms if you are not able to accept yourself as a loving person. You are lovable and you deserve to receive love. Reiki can help you to achieve self-love when you are open to giving to yourself in this way. It can teach you how to love and nurture yourself more fully, preparing you to accept whatever life brings you: a lover or soulmate, a baby, a new project to undertake, or something else entirely.

Reiki During Pregnancy

Reiki can be beneficial for all age groups, even for those who are not yet born. Pregnant women who are attuned to Reiki can extend love to their unborn children by laying their hands on their belly and allowing Reiki energies to be taken in by their babies.

Some Reiki practitioners feel that if a woman is attuned to Reiki during her pregnancy, her baby is also attuned to the energies. What a wonderful gift to offer your child before its birthday!

It is perfectly safe for a pregnant woman to have a full-body Reiki treatment. Reiki will flow to both mother and child. What a bargain, getting two treatments for the price of one.

Reiki and Children

Reiki's gentle and noninvasive nature is also perfect for treating the ills and upsets of young children. Children are extremely receptive to Reiki's positive effects and will normally welcome Reiki without any apprehension, especially when they receive treatments from their parents.

Reiki treatments are to be given to children much in the same manner as they are given to adults. The basic hand placements are the same. However, the treatment will not last as long. Reiki energies travel swiftly through a child's body—unlike adults, children don't yet have years of accumulated toxins or blockages that tend to slow down the treatment process. If the child becomes restless or fidgety when receiving Reiki, the treatment should be ended. Children will often instinctively sit up and move away from the Reiki practitioner when they feel they have had enough.

Attuning Children

Babies and toddlers can be attuned to Reiki, but they are not mature enough to learn how to practice it. Children younger than five years of age lack the comprehension skills to understand the concepts of Reiki.

Most children between the ages of five and twelve have the ability to learn Reiki and can be attuned to the first level. One or two Reiki attunements may be all that are needed to attune children to Reiki Level I. Traditionally, four attunements are required for adults. Also, young children should not be expected to sit through a full day or even a half day of Reiki instruction, since their attention spans are shorter. Teachers should attune the child and give him only basic instructions. Afterward, it is appropriate for the parent to carefully guide and assist the child in the use of Reiki in the home. For this reason, the only children who should be attuned to Reiki are those with a parent or other adult in the home who is an experienced practitioner of Reiki.

REIKI REFLECTIONS

Children should be cautioned not to force their Reiki hands or energies upon classmates who may not understand or appreciate what they are attempting to do. Instead, have children focus on practicing Reiki at home. It is essential that your child first be ready for Reiki. Children enjoy giving Reiki to their dolls and stuffed animals, as well as to their pets and siblings.

If you are considering having your child attuned, it is a good idea to arrange a time for the child and teacher to meet with each other before the day of attunement arrives. Preferably, this meeting would take place in the same environment where the class would be held. Look to see that your child is comfortable and at ease with both the teacher and the environment. If you notice that your child shows fear or appears resistant in any way, you should hold off on scheduling a class.

Reiki and Pets

Many people today look for a holistic approach to treating illnesses in their animal companions. Animal lovers are sensitive to their pets' illnesses. Likewise, pets can be sensitive to the sufferings of their caregivers. Many dogs and cats absorb Reiki energies more quickly than humans. This could simply be the result of their size (at least for most cats and small- to medium-sized dog breeds), but more likely it is because they inherently understand what Reiki is. Most cats and dogs will accept the energies they need and allow you to place your hands on them freely. When they have had enough, they will simply walk away. A full treatment could be over in five minutes. Treatments seldom last more than twenty minutes.

You can give Reiki to your pets by touching, stroking, or patting them. Reiki can also be sent to animals through distance healing if they are skittish or confused by your touch—or if you are allergic to an animal's fur or dander. Absentia healing is a must for treating nondomestic animals such as terrestrial wildlife, zoo animals, and aquatic creatures.

Here is how Reiki can help your pet:

- It accelerates the healing of physical injuries.
- It promotes peace and calmness.
- It treats trauma from accidents or surgery, nervousness, and fear.
- It reduces stress and suffering.
- It helps promote bonding between animal and pet owner.
- It treats behavioral problems: chewing, biting, scratching, excessive barking, and so on.

- It offers a comforting transitional energy when it is time for your pet to depart from this world.

It's Good for Grandma, Too!

Reiki is suitable for people of all ages, but because of Reiki's pain management capabilities, seniors especially welcome it—probably because it offers help in alleviating the aches and pains associated with aging.

Reiki's effectiveness varies from person to person. Some ailments respond more favorably to Reiki than others. Also, some people are more receptive to Reiki. Many seniors have come to the realization that they can no longer do everything for themselves. They have also learned that life can be easier if they stop resisting help when and where it is offered. Because of their diminished physical or mental capabilities, many older adults have been forced to depend on others in order for their needs to be met. As a result, they are normally more readily accepting of Reiki's assistance.

REIKI REFLECTIONS

Energy medicine such as Reiki is recognized as both a beneficial and complementary therapy to conventional medicine helpful in pain management.

Reiki does not prejudice or favor anyone by age, gender, or species. You and all members of your family (grandparents, parents, aunts, uncles, spouse, cousins, siblings, pets, and so on—even your plants) can benefit from Reiki. What better reason could there be to learn Reiki than having the ability to share it with those you love?

PART 5

EXPLORING REIKI

*In wisdom gathered over time I have found that
every experience is a form of exploration.*

Ansel Adams

In this part, you'll further explore the more technical aspects of Reiki, such as learning about the various levels of training, how you can become certified, and what you can expect to experience during these attunement sessions and how to prepare.

Next, you'll delve more deeply into the meaning and use of the five main Reiki symbols, their power, and how to use them in meditation. Then, you'll also discover more about the various Reiki systems that have arisen over the years and how they have sprung from a common source.

Finally, you'll have a chance to learn more about nontraditional forms of Reiki, what Reiki is not, how it's different from other healing modalities, how to use it with other healing practices, and how to stay on the Reiki path.

CHAPTER 14

REIKI LEVELS OF TRAINING

Health is a state of body. Wellness is a state of being.

Jason Stanford

IN THIS CHAPTER, you'll learn more about the three levels of basic training in Usui Reiki: Level I, Level II, and Level III. At the highest level, you may become a Reiki Master/Teacher, but as this chapter discusses, being certified in the highest level does not necessarily reflect superior knowledge. It is through the continued practice of Reiki that one becomes proficient. The Level I practitioner who uses Reiki daily will be more aware of how Reiki works than a Level III Reiki Master/Teacher who seldom conducts treatments.

Getting Certified

The Reiki student is attuned to Reiki during her classroom session through an initiation ceremony that is traditionally passed down from Master (teacher) to student. The attunement process is what makes Reiki stand apart from other types of healing-touch systems. Although other healing arts may use hand placements, only Reiki has the wonderful benefit of the attunement process. At each level of attunement, Reiki certificates are awarded to students at the end of the class.

Each Reiki Master/Teacher uses her own methodology in teaching Reiki classes. Traditionally, each level of Reiki was taught separately. A period of weeks, months, or even years could pass before the Reiki student could go on to the next level. This afforded students time to learn how to use each level proficiently before advancing to the next one. Some Reiki teachers remain true to this tradition. These teachers will only accept a student in their Reiki Level II and Reiki Level III classes when they feel that the student has assimilated the teachings of Level I and Level II, respectively. Not all teachers adhere to this tradition, however.

Today, you can find almost any combination of Reiki levels taught during one class session. A weekend class could offer both Levels I and II, or even all three levels. The material covered and instructions given may vary somewhat from one classroom to another, but as long as the teacher passes attunements to her students, Reiki will become a part of these students forever.

Once Reiki is awakened within you through the attunement ceremony, your journey as a Reiki practitioner begins.

Usui Reiki Level I

Level I is the introductory class to Usui Reiki. In this class, students will receive one, two, or four attunements. The students will learn the history of Reiki, either through listening to the oral tradition or by receiving written handouts that they can take home afterward to read at their leisure. Students will also learn (or review) basic hand placements for giving self-treatments and for treating others. First, the students usually conduct a full-body self-treatment. Then, they may pair off to give and receive a treatment, or the class will participate as a whole in group Reiki treatments.

REIKI REFLECTIONS

If you have a friend or a relative who shares your interest in Reiki, the two of you may prefer to sign up for a Reiki class together. Using Reiki during and after the class, the two of you will be able to lovingly support one another as you progress with Reiki.

Signing Up for Class

There are a few things to keep in mind when preparing to take your first Reiki class. First, you may be asked to send full payment or a partial deposit a few days or weeks in advance to reserve your place in the class. Often classes are held in people's homes, where the lack of space might limit class size. Attending a class with only a small number of students, perhaps five or less, can be beneficial in allowing more one-on-one attention between the teacher and students, more time for all of your questions to be answered, and so on. Many individuals who are drawn to learn Reiki are passionate and loving people. Lifetime friendships are likely to develop among the people you will meet in your Reiki classes.

Don't be late for class. Not only does it show poor manners, but it will also inconvenience the teacher by disrupting his well-planned schedule. In such a circumstance, the teacher might either choose to start the class without you, forcing him to help you get caught up later on, or make everyone wait for your arrival before beginning the class, thus possibly inconveniencing other members of the class as well.

Preparing for Class

Wear comfortable clothing made of natural fibers such as cotton, wool, or silk. Some teachers ask that you wear all white when getting your Level I and Level II attunements. They will usually specify this prior to class. Do not wear nylon stockings or any other restrictive types of garments. And don't forget to eat a good breakfast or meal beforehand!

If you are attending a class that will be held out of town, consider reserving a room at a local hotel for an overnight stay following your day in class. You will be receiving your attunements and may be participating in three or more full-body treatments. This amounts to a lot of ki energies running through your body.

REIKI REFLECTIONS

Unless you give plenty of advance notice to your Reiki teacher, don't expect a prepayment or deposit to be refunded if you choose to cancel your class. Advance notice will allow the teacher sufficient time to locate and arrange for another student to take your place.

Attunements by themselves have been known to overwhelm students who are not accustomed to operating on a full tank of energy. Unless you have done some type of energy work prior to your introduction to Reiki, you won't really know how your body will react to that first blast of Reiki energies that surge through it. Some people experience drowsiness or exhaustion, while others feel exhilaration or a sense of loftiness. Some students have reported a sort of buzzing sensation, feeling as if an electric vibrator is running on a high setting right inside their bodies.

Perhaps none of these examples will be representative of your own experience, but should any of them occur, driving home after the class is not a great idea. Even if you believe yourself to be capable of driving, pack an overnight bag to keep in the car with you just in case you do decide later to stop along the way home and spend the night in a motel or with a friend.

Basic Class Overview—Reiki Level I

Usually, a basic Reiki Level I class will take somewhere between eight and sixteen hours. Some teachers hold Reiki Level I classes over a two-day period (usually the weekend), while other teachers divide Level I Reiki into two sessions that are held over two consecutive weekends. What follows is a sample syllabus for an eight-hour Reiki Level I class.

Class Schedule

The class will begin at 9:00 A.M. and go on until 6:00 P.M., including a one-hour break for lunch.

Classroom Introductions

At the beginning of the class, before instruction gets underway, you have a brief period of time to learn your classmates' names and talk informally with your instructor. You may be asked to share something about yourself with the class. For instance, your instructor may ask all the students to state why they are taking the class and what expectations they have, if any.

Class Overview

At the beginning of the class, the teacher may choose to give a formal lecture on Reiki or to facilitate a class discussion about it. Traditionally, this is the time when the "story of Reiki" is told. The teacher also tells the students what to expect during the class sessions and prompts them to ask any questions they might have before he passes the attunements and teaches the basic hand placements.

Reiki Attunements

The teacher gives basic instructions about how and when attunements are passed. For an all-day class, the passing of attunements could be divided into four short sessions. For example, you might receive two attunements in the morning and two more attunements in the afternoon.

Self-Treatment Instructions

Students are taught the basic hand placements that are used for a full-body self-treatment. Each member of the class gives himself a self-treatment while the teacher supervises.

Instructions for Treating Others

Students are taught the basic hand placements for treating others. To learn, the students practice in pairs, or the teacher may choose to divide them into small groups. Each student should give at least one full-body treatment to another person and receive at least one full-body treatment from someone else.

End of Class

At the end of the class session, you are awarded a certificate for completion of Usui Reiki Level I. Congratulations!

Usui Reiki Level II

Reiki Level II is a continuation of Level I. This level offers the students increased power and the ability to give absentia, or distance, Reiki treatments. In the Reiki Level II class, the teacher will reveal to the students the first three Reiki symbols and how they can be used in Reiki treatments. In addition to learning the symbols' meanings and practicing drawing them onto paper, the students will learn how to use the symbols to enhance hands-on sessions and for their absentia treatments.

Traditionally, Reiki Level II classes are not available to everyone. Not only does the student need to be already certified as a Reiki Level I practitioner, the instructor must sense that the student is ready to move forward to the next level. Teaching second-level or third-level Reiki to a person who isn't psychologically or emotionally ready for it, or who is interested in learning Reiki simply for the money or prestige, would be a disservice to Reiki, to the student, and to the teacher.

Here are a few questions the Reiki Level I practitioner should ask herself before considering going on to Reiki Level II:

- Am I ready for this next step?
- Can I feel Reiki sensations in my palms?
- Do I have a general understanding of Reiki?
- Am I using Reiki on a regular basis?
- What are my reasons for wanting to move on to Reiki Level II?

Basic Class Overview—Reiki Level II

A Reiki Level II class takes approximately six hours to complete and is normally taught in two three-hour sessions, with a break between sessions. It could also be taught in one morning and an afternoon, but it is preferable to teach this class on a weekend, over a two-day period. The following is a sample syllabus for a six-hour Reiki Level II class.

Class Schedule
Friday: 7:00 P.M. until 10:00 P.M. Saturday: 9:00 A.M. until noon.

Introduction Period
Students are given a few minutes to meet and socialize. Typically, students will discuss their individual experiences as Reiki Level I practitioners and their reasons for deciding to take Reiki Level II.

Reiki Level I Review
The teacher gives a brief review of Reiki Level I, and then students have the opportunity to ask any questions they have concerning Level I and anything else they want to know before they go on to Level II.

Reiki Attunement Rite
Next, the first of two attunements is passed to the students.

Reiki Symbols
The students are introduced to three distinct Reiki symbols (Power, Connection, and Harmony). Students learn how to precisely draw these symbols. They also learn about the power of the symbols and how to pronounce their names and spell them properly. Sketchpads are provided for students to use to practice drawing the symbols as they are taught.

Homework Assignment
The Reiki symbols are to be memorized by Saturday morning's class.

Saturday Morning Exam
Students are tested to make sure they can draw the Reiki symbols from memory, recite the symbols' names using correct pronunciations, and know the powers of each symbol.

Reiki Attunement Rite

Then, the second attunement is passed to the students.

Working and Playing with the Symbols

Students learn the absentia Reiki formula and practice sending Reiki treatments to others. The remainder of the class is used to further explore the Reiki symbols. The class may conduct exercises and play games that involve the symbols.

At first you might find a Reiki Level II class to be reminiscent of both an art class and a kindergarten class rolled into one. This is because you get to hug teddy bears and draw pictures on art paper with colorful crayons. You might have to be quick to get your hands on the purple crayon before another classmate beats you to it: Purple is said to naturally carry the vibration of Reiki. That's why it helps to go to your class fully prepared. Have your own purple marker or crayon tucked inside your pocket or purse. You might also be requested to paint imaginary symbols in the air with your hands. For exercises such as these, Reiki Level II energies will awaken the imaginative powers of the innocent child within you.

REIKI REFLECTIONS

Reiki Level II is a fun class to take. The energy level in the classroom is both warm and playful. Remember, everyone in the class is already a Reiki practitioner, so the overall vibes are going to be great. The memorization requirement for learning the symbols can feel quite challenging and even a bit stressful for some, but the symbols really are not that difficult to learn. Relax and enjoy!

End of Class

The class ends with a brief question-and-answer period. You are awarded a certificate for completion of Usui Reiki Level II. Congratulations!

Usui Reiki Level III

How are Reiki III practitioners different from Reiki Masters? Basically, Reiki Level III is the Reiki Master Level of attunement. Here are the basic distinctions:

- Reiki Level III—Title of practitioner who has received the Reiki Master Level attunement.
- Reiki Master—Title of practitioner who has received the Reiki Master Level attunement *and* has been shown the Master symbol.
- Reiki Master/Teacher—Title of practitioner who has received the Reiki Master Level attunement, has been shown the Master symbol, *and* has been taught how to pass attunements to others.

However, these distinctions are somewhat muddied because the title of "Reiki Master" is routinely used by all three categories of practitioners defined in this list. Many Master/Teacher practitioners will certify as a "Reiki Master" anyone who has received the Master Level attunement, regardless of whether or not she has been given the Master symbol, has learned how to pass attunements, or has received instructions on how to conduct Reiki classes.

When you make the decision to advance from Reiki Level II, it is crucial that you interview several teachers in order to find out what type of training you would receive from them. Also, ask yourself what your motives are for seeking advancement. Are you interested in becoming a teacher and passing on attunements to students? Or are you only trying to receive the Master Level attunement? Unfortunately, some students seek out Master certification only for the sake of title or prestige.

Usui Reiki Master Level

Going through the process of becoming a Reiki Master/Teacher is an intense healing experience on a very personal level. Reiki, as you will learn from going through Reiki Level I and Reiki Level II, brings about balance in your life. Graduation from a Reiki Master Level class does not close the chapter on learning Reiki. Reiki will become an integral part of your life, and learning more about it will continue throughout your lifetime as you use it. The following is a sample syllabus for a Reiki Master/Teacher Level class.

Forty Classroom Hours

Students in a Reiki Master/Teacher Level class meet with their instructor for eight-hour class sessions once a week for five weeks. Throughout the course of five weeks, students are instructed to give themselves a full-body self-treatment each day.

First Week

Students and teacher write out goals they hope to achieve in the class. These goals are read out loud every time the class meets. The teacher will present a brief lecture that details the content of the five-week course. Students will be instructed to keep a journal in which they record in detail their personal experiences in the class as well as outside of the classroom. These "experience stories" will be used in their own classes when they start teaching Reiki.

During the class, the teacher will also pass the Master Level attunement to the students and will teach them the Master and Completion symbols. The teacher might end with the following homework assignment: Study the history of Reiki. Write down your experience stories. Study the instruction handouts for passing the first and second attunements for Reiki Level I.

Second Week

The teacher reads aloud the class's goals. Students may read their personal goals aloud if they choose. Class size may not allow time for every student to read his goals. Students share their experience stories with the teacher and their classmates. The students present the oral history of Dr. Mikao Usui. New experiences since receiving Reiki Master attunement are discussed.

The students learn how to conduct Reiki Level I classes and review how to pass the first and second attunements for Reiki Level I. The following would be assigned for homework: Continue to add experience stories to your list. Review the history of Reiki. Practice the attunement process. Study the instruction handouts for passing the third and fourth attunements for Reiki Level I. Memorize all Reiki symbols, including the Master and Completion symbols.

Third Week

Again, the teacher reviews the goals by reading them out loud, and students share their experience stories. Then, students present the oral history of Dr. Hayashi, a student of Usui who played a major role in the development of Reiki in the western world.

Students review how to pass the third and fourth attunements for Reiki Level I. The Reiki Level II class structure is discussed. Students are tested on all of the symbols—how to draw, pronounce, and interpret them. As a homework assignment, students may be required to study instructional handouts on passing attunements for Reiki Level II and to review the history of Reiki.

Fourth Week

After the overview of the class goals and sharing experience stories, students present the oral history of Mrs. Hawayo Takata. Then, students go over how to pass attunements for Reiki Level II. The Reiki Level II class structure is also reviewed. Classroom and Reiki Master ethics are discussed. The homework assignment is to study instructional handouts for passing Master Level attunements.

Fifth Week

The last class begins in the usual manner, with the reading of goals, followed by students sharing their experience stories. Then, students go over how to pass attunements for the Reiki Master Level and the class structure of the Reiki Master Level class.

End of Class

The class ends with a brief question-and-answer period. You are awarded a certificate for completion of the Usui Reiki Master Level. Congratulations!

REIKI REFLECTIONS

At the end of the Reiki Level III class, students review passing attunements for all levels. Additional classes are scheduled for any students who feel that they may need more instruction.

What It All Means

Certifications in the various levels of Reiki are paper documents noting participation and accomplishment in classroom studies. In the end, the surest way to develop a true mastering of Reiki is through practicing it routinely, applying the five Reiki principles, and involving Reiki in every aspect of your daily life.

Reiki Level I is the awakening. Reiki Level II is intended to increase the students' power and to teach them how to assist others by learning how to do distance healings. Reiki III and Master Levels are intended to teach students the skills needed to teach and pass attunements to others. A distinctive attunement ritual is passed from teacher to student at each level.

CHAPTER 15

REIKI SYMBOLS

Listen to your intuition. It will tell you everything you need to know.

Anthony J. D'Angelo

FIVE SYMBOLS ARE USED in the Usui Reiki attunement process. Four of these symbols are also used in conducting both hands-on and absentia treatments. Much mystery surrounds the Reiki symbols because of the tradition to honor their sacredness and to guard them from the eyes of non-practitioners. However, since they are instantly available on the Internet, this secrecy is no longer possible to maintain, which is why the symbols are pictured in Chapter 8. But, as you'll learn in this chapter, simply knowing what the symbol looks like—or being able to draw it—is not what activates its power. You must be attuned in order to use the symbols effectively.

In this chapter, you'll learn about the development, definitions, purposes, and methods of using the Reiki symbols, and you'll see why they are the subjects of great interest and discussion.

The Power of a Symbol

Through Hawayo Takata's Reiki stories, her students were taught that the Reiki symbols were revealed to Dr. Mikao Usui through spiritual enlightenment on the twenty-first day of his meditation fast on Mount Kurama. According to Takata, Usui had recognized these symbols from his studies of the ancient Sanskrit writings kept in the monastery's libraries, but before his spiritual awakening on the mountain, he supposedly had no understanding of the meanings or the purpose of these symbols.

However, no definite proof that Usui actually reviewed or studied any Sanskrit documents has ever come to light. Also, the Reiki symbols employed by Usui are formulated from Chinese and Japanese kanji characters, not Sanskrit lettering. Usui either developed the Reiki symbols on his own, or he may have translated them from the ethereal knowledge revealed to him on the mountain by using his own written language, Japanese kanji.

Japanese Kanji

Kanji are modified Chinese characters, originally imported from China. In addition to its use of kanji, the Japanese writing system also relies on hiragana and katakana, alphabetic systems that represent various sounds, as opposed to ideas or words.

For the Japanese, a handwritten kanji is a character equivalent to a written letter, word, or phrase in Western handwriting. Kanji characters are pictograms that represent ideas or words, rather than merely alphabetic letters or syllables of words that you would sound out in order to read. Whereas the word "Reiki" consists of five letters in the English alphabet, in Japanese writings Reiki is pictured as a "kanji-pair." In other words, Reiki is represented by two individual kanji symbols, often drawn one on top of the other. The top symbol is rei, meaning "universal life," and the lower symbol is ki, meaning "energy."

Before the invention of typewriters and computers with Japanese fonts, the Japanese wrote their characters with a paintbrush or pen. There are many versions of "Reiki kanji," mainly because of the differences in people's handwriting styles.

1. sacred ground
2. established rule
3. chill; cold weather
4. electrical excitation
5. aura
6. healing method

The Five Reiki Symbols

However he derived them, Usui used the five Reiki symbols as practical teaching tools for his students—the symbols were meant to assist the students in focusing and holding intention while giving treatments and passing attunements.

FIVE TRADITIONAL REIKI SYMBOLS

Japanese Name	English Name	Intention	Purposes
Cho Ku Rei	Power symbol	Light switch	Manifestation; increased power; accelerated healing; healing catalyst
Sei Hei Ki	Harmony symbol	Purification	Cleansing; protection; mental and emotional healing
Hon Sha Ze Sho Nen	Connection symbol	Timelessness	Distance healing; past/present/future; healing karma; spiritual connection
Dai Ko Myo	Master symbol	Enlightenment	Empowerment; soul healing; oneness
Raku	Completion symbol	Grounding	Kundalini healing; hara connection; chakra alignment

Imagery Is a Universal Language

Energy, in its purest essence, does not possess form, nor is it visually identifiable. However, in the physical world in which we live, the concept of visualizing or touching a structured energy form is often easier to comprehend than visualizing manipulation of shapeless or invisible energy. Usui's symbols became visual representations of "all that Reiki is." Usui understood that Reiki is a universal energy. He not only was able to give the symbols to his students as healing tools, but through graphic images, he managed to give Reiki its own universal language.

Imagery truly is a universal language—eye candy for our visual pleasure. Everyday pictures, icons, and symbols are used in our communications to represent our ideas and inspirations. When they are viewed, certain images can signify clear-cut meanings. Consider a glowing light bulb to symbolize a bright idea, the skull and crossbones to warn of poisonous contents, a red heart to indicate love, and the four-leaf clover to suggest good fortune. When we see these easily recognizable images, their associated meanings come to our minds instantly.

When practitioners use Reiki symbols regularly, they soon learn that the power is not in the symbols themselves but in the purposes and intentions that the symbols represent and solidify.

Traditional Secrecy

As stated previously, Reiki students are introduced to the first three symbols after they are attuned to Reiki Level II, and those who go on to the Reiki Master/Teacher Level are taught the two remaining symbols. An introduction to Reiki symbols includes learning how to draw them and instruction as to what they mean and how they may be used in Reiki.

Traditionally, any drawings of the Reiki symbols on paper were burned in a ritual at the end of the classes. Sometimes this ritual would be a part of the class. At other times the teacher would perform a private ritual, burning the drawings after the students were gone. Modern teachers who still honor the tradition of keeping the symbols private will either burn the drawings or use a paper shredder so that the paper waste can later be recycled. Other teachers see no harm in allowing students to keep their classroom drawings and may even provide pre-drawn diagrams in handouts that the students can keep for future reference.

REIKI REFLECTIONS

Whenever any Reiki symbol is to be used, the practitioner recites it three times. This may be done aloud or mentally as the practitioner traces the symbol in the air over the recipient's body.

Today, diagrams of the Reiki symbols can be readily found printed in books and displayed on the Internet, so true secrecy is no longer possible.

Cho Ku Rei—the Power Symbol

The Reiki Power symbol is the first symbol presented to Reiki initiates and is the most commonly used Reiki symbol. In fact, it is used more often than all of the other symbols combined. See Figure 8.1.

Reiki practitioners use the Cho Ku Rei symbol by itself or in combination with the other symbols. When conducting an absentia treatment, using two Power symbols as energetic bookends with a Connection symbol sandwiched in between creates a power-packed vacuum space that will travel at lightning speed. When the treatment is delivered, the results can be immediate and far-reaching.

From a Visual Perspective

When you draw the symbols on paper, they will appear flat and lifeless. However, if you draw them in the air, they evolve into three-dimensional animated images. It is as if the ki energies breathe life into them. The symbols will float in the air as if they are hanging from a mobile. They will shrink and enlarge and even change colors. The symbols will float across the room where you sit while conducting a full-body treatment on a client. From there you will manipulate the symbols either mentally or with your hands, as needed.

Purrs Like a Kitten

The Power symbol is a wonderful catalyst for the healing process. If you have ever held a purring kitten, you will understand the "motor" vibration associated with the Cho Ku Rei. There is an underlying current, or charge, that resides in the core of the coil of this symbol. The strength of this charge may be subtle at times and revved up high at other times, but even though the energy embedded within the symbol may cool down or unwind, it always maintains a constant pulse.

You can draw the Cho Ku Rei with as many spiral movements as you feel are appropriate for the situation at hand. Printed diagrams of the Cho Ku Rei normally show two-and-a-half coils, but you can draw the Cho Ku Rei with as many coils as you like. Don't worry about winding up any coil too tightly, and be sure to draw the coils, or spirals, in a counterclockwise direction.

Metaphysical Multiplier

The primary intention of using the Cho Ku Rei is to increase power. This is why it is praised for its manifestation power; it is a metaphysical multiplier. No matter what aspect of your life you desire to increase, Reiki's Power symbol is an intention tool that can help bring it to fruition. There are many areas in your life that can benefit from the boost of energy provided by the Cho Ku Rei. Listed here are just some of the effects this symbol can have:

- Bolster self-confidence
- Increase cash flow
- Expand time
- Actualize dreams
- Intensify creativity
- Boost immune system
- Promote spiritual growth
- Magnify happiness

Sei Hei Ki—the Harmony Symbol

The Reiki Harmony symbol is the second symbol Reiki initiates learn in their Level II class. This symbol is used as a purification tool and is also helpful to anyone dealing with emotional or mental disturbances. This is the symbol that assists a person who is trying to break a simple bad habit or overcome the grip of a serious physiological or mental addiction. See Fig. 8.2.

Like a Fire-Breathing Dragon

The Sei Hei Ki looks remarkably like a cartoon dragon. Cartoon dragons are not to be feared. Rather, they should be understood and enjoyed as friendly and courageous beings.

Nevertheless, the Reiki dragon is up to the challenge when faced with fighting off adversity. Although the symbol does not show the dragon's fiery breath, you can easily add it in your imagination. The fire essence within the Sei Hei Ki serves as a purification flame. It scorches addictions and expels negative energies, leaving nothing but smoldering ashes upon the ground, allowing the rebirth of energy in its purest form.

A Personal Bodyguard

In addition to its label as the Harmony symbol, the Sei Hei Ki is also often named the Protection symbol. In its protective capacity, the Sei Hei Ki can be used as an antiseptic "ointment" before, during, and after surgery. It can also be applied as a protective shield prior to and following purification ceremonies or whenever menacing energies have been removed from a person's auric field or physical body.

Sei Hei Ki can be used in prayer mantras when asking for personal protection and safe travel conditions before driving, flying, taking a vacation cruise, and so on. The Sei Hei Ki symbol can be placed inside packages as additional insurance for their safe delivery before dropping them off at the post office. This Protection symbol can even be placed in condoms as an extra precaution before indulging in sex.

As with all protective measures, there is no guarantee that using the Sei Hei Ki will be 100 percent effective. If it's in the cards, a traffic accident or pregnancy could still occur, no matter how many precautions have been taken. However, using the Sei Hei Ki as a cautionary intention in your day-to-day existence is recommended. After all, would you go out without wearing an overcoat if a heavy rainstorm were in the forecast? Of course, you wouldn't. The Sei Hei Ki is an added protective covering to help you weather the stormy elements of life.

Hon Sha Ze Sho Nen—the Connection Symbol

The Reiki Connection symbol is the third symbol taught to Reiki initiates. The Hon Sha Ze Sho Nen is best known for its use in distance, or absentia, treatments. This symbol has a long reach; it extends beyond time and space. This symbol is also called the Pagoda because of its tower-like appearance—multiple kanji characters are used to create it. More variations have been shown of this symbol than of any of the other Reiki symbols. See Fig. 8.3.

From a visual point of view, the Hon Sha Ze Sho Nen is a cosmic shape-shifter. This symbol is extremely adaptable and feels elastic when you work with it. Its form collapses and stretches, as needed, in any application. More so than the other symbols, the Hon Sha Ze Sho Nen seems to exhibit extra flexibility.

REIKI REFLECTIONS

All of the Reiki symbols are flexible. Working with these symbols could be described as handling modeling clay. Clay sculptures express what the artist feels. In this same way, the Reiki symbols emulate intentions put forth by the Reiki practitioner.

Absentia Treatments

The Hon Sha Ze Sho Nen is always used in transmitting absentia, or distance, treatments. It possesses the power of telepathy and is comparable to the electrical wiring that connects telegraph operators on each end of a communication.

Inner-Child Therapy

The Hon Sha Ze Sho Nen also can assist you in making a connection with your inner child. Unresolved childhood traumas and issues tend to get buried inside our subconscious minds, contributing to our adult fears and concerns. Reiki treatments can bring about balance, and will sometimes bring these issues to the surface for healing. When you encounter hurtful memories that were formerly locked up inside a recipient but are suddenly beginning to surface, it is appropriate to apply this symbol to assist the ki movement toward balance and healing.

Akashic Records

The Connection symbol serves as the key to accessing information recorded in the Akashic Records. This information is included for individuals who believe in reincarnation. If you believe that you have lived many lifetimes, you probably also believe that when you entered your current incarnation, you brought in talents and knowledge that you attained during previous incarnations. Also, any emotional backlash from pains or sufferings in past lives that were not completely healed would also have been carried into this life at birth.

One school of thought teaches the belief that all of our lifetimes (past, present, and future) are being lived out simultaneously in different dimensions. The Hon Sha Ze Sho Nen symbol can extend to past and future lives and treat all dis-eases from all of our lifetimes. Applying Reiki to ailments that originated in previous lifetimes will treat the physical dis-ease during that lifetime, and as a bonus, will also treat any lingering emotional repercussions that were carried over into the present lifetime.

When visualizing the Reiki symbols, pay attention to whether or not they appear balanced. A symbol that appears askew is signaling an imbalance. For example, if you're conducting a distance treatment and the Cho Ku Rei appears lopsided, it could mean that the recipient's personal power is diminished. Or, if the Sei Hei Ki appears squashed, it could indicate disharmony. In these cases, ask your Reiki guides to bring balance to the misaligned symbol before sending it off to the recipient.

Dai Ko Myo—the Master Symbol

The Master symbol is possibly the single most coveted Reiki symbol by first- and second-degree practitioners. This is because most people are achievement-oriented. We want to earn the highest badge or be awarded the grandest trophy. See Fig. 8.4.

The energy represented by the Reiki Master symbol is powerful. It represents all that is Reiki, including love and personal empowerment. This is why the Master symbol is included in all levels of attunement. All levels of Reiki practitioners receive the Dai Ko Myo symbol from their teacher through the attunement ritual. It is not an exclusive energy available only to some people; Dai Ko Myo love energy is accessible to everyone.

Being attuned to Reiki Master Level and knowing how to draw the Master symbol are required for teachers in order for them to be able to attune others. But, aside from that, the symbol is seldom, if ever, used. The symbol can be drawn or visualized in healings, but the essence of this symbol is already in the energy of Reiki itself. Probably the only time it might be called upon is whenever you are treating someone who is struggling with self-love.

Raku—the Completion Symbol

The last Reiki symbol in the Usui Reiki system is the Raku. This symbol is used only in the final stage of the attunement ritual in order to separate the teacher's aura from the student's aura. Its energy is very forceful and should carefully be placed between the two individuals. See Fig. 8.5.

Aside from being used to separate the auras and align the student's chakras, the Raku has no other use in Reiki. Its appearance is that of a sharp zigzag image that resembles a lightning bolt. The Raku is drawn from top to bottom. An alternate Raku symbol, occasionally used by nontraditional Reiki Masters, resembles a winding snake and represents kundalini energy.

Meditation and Reiki Symbols

Each symbol carries its own unique energy and has distinct purposes. Once you learn a symbol, spend some time with it individually in order to form a close relationship with it. The symbols are wonderful healing tools, but trying to use them without knowing their full potential or understanding how or when to utilize them will diminish your awareness of the healing process. Meditate on each symbol individually and take note of any sensations and thoughts that surface.

The Reiki symbols are very beautiful, but they have no power by themselves. They are merely visual representations of all that Reiki has to offer. The symbols serve as tools to assist Reiki practitioners when practitioners shape their healing intentions during treatments for themselves and others. Each practitioner develops her own unique relationship with the symbols.

CHAPTER 16

REIKI SYSTEMS

The greatest mistake in the treatment of diseases is that there are physicians for the body and physicians for the soul, although the two cannot be separated.

Plato

MANY VARIATIONS OF REIKI have been developed since Dr. Usui first made his discovery, and new versions of Reiki continue to evolve today. In this chapter, you'll learn a bit more about each of these—how they came about, their similarities, and their differences. Each system offers its own unique twist to the simple art of Reiki. Some of the variant systems imply mysterious or metaphysical origins. Several of these methodologies claim to have made use of newly created or rediscovered traditional Reiki systems that are somehow superior to the original documented teachings. By spending some time learning about them, you can make your own decision.

A Variety of Systems

Once Hawayo Takata introduced Reiki to the West, her established tradition of passing down information about Reiki from teacher to student through spoken word, rather than written text, allowed leeway for modifications through interpretational differences. The history of Reiki took on different flavorings, depending on how each teacher retold the stories to help students better understand and remember the teachings.

The Reiki kanji symbols used in passing attunements and distance healing were written down on paper only for a brief time during instruction in order to facilitate memorization during instruction. After memorization, the papers were destroyed to keep the symbols secret. Relying on memory alone to preserve the teachings of Reiki left plenty of room for mistakes to enter in and for blatant deviations from the original materials to become incorporated into the works.

After Hawayo Takata's death (in 1980), a major split occurred among the twenty-two Masters she had initiated, when two individuals declared themselves to be Hawayo Takata's successors. Phyllis Lei Furumoto, granddaughter of Hawayo Takata, proclaimed she was the lineage bearer and Grand Master of Reiki. In 1983, Furumoto helped to organize the Reiki Alliance.

For her part, Dr. Barbara Ray states she is Takata's successor, which gives her the distinction of being the Holder of the Intact Master Keys of Reiki. The succession of Holders of the Intact Master Keys of Reiki, according to Dr. Ray, goes like this:

1. Dr. Mikao Usui
2. Dr. Jujiro (Chujiro) Hayashi
3. Hawayo Takata
4. Dr. Barbara Ray

In addition to this split, many other students branched out from the original teaching and developed their own systems of practicing and teaching Reiki.

The Original Systems

Dr. Mikao Usui is internationally recognized as the founder of Reiki. His findings and experiences of using Universal Life Energy for healing were passed down to others. Usui's teachings remain the foundation of most of the Reiki systems used today.

Usui Reiki Ryoho, as it originated from Mikao Usui, is still practiced in Japan. It teaches spiritual development and self-healing through empowerments and meditations. These empowerments, such as Reiju, are used instead of the attunements in order to open and clear the Reiki passageways within the initiates.

Usui Shiki Ryoho

The Usui Shiki Ryoho system emerged from the Usui-Hayashi lineage. This is the traditional Usui System of Natural Healing that made its way to the United States from Japan through the teachings of Mrs. Hawayo Takata. The primary principles taught in this book are based on the fundamental teachings of this system, its principles, attunements, symbols, and hand placements.

Raku Kei Reiki

Arthur Robertson developed Raku Kei Reiki. He designed this system to enhance the Reiki experience. Arthur Robertson's lineage is Mikao Usui–Chujiro Hayashi–Hawayo Takata–Iris Ishikuro.

Raku Kei Reiki was a precursor to Usui/Tibetan Reiki, Vajra Reiki, Karuna Reiki, and Tera Mai Reiki. Raku Kei incorporates the Hui Yin, the Breath of the Fire Dragon, kundalini breathing, and other Tibetan practices and symbolism.

Usui/Tibetan Reiki

Usui/Tibetan Reiki combines Usui Shiki Ryoho Reiki, Raku Kei Reiki, and Advanced Reiki Training (ART). This system, popularized by William Lee Rand and Diane Stein, has four levels of training: Reiki I, II, IIIa, and III/Master. Level IIIa of this system, also referred to as ART, consists of a variety of add-on techniques such as the use of crystal grids, guides, healing attunement, psychic surgery, meditations, and Tibetan symbols.

Trademarked Systems

In 1997, Phyllis Lei Furumoto attempted to trademark the word "Reiki," along with the terms "Usui Shiki Ryoho" and "Usui System." Her attempts failed. However, specialized Reiki systems, such as Tera Mai and Karuna Reiki, have successfully been trademarked, as their inceptions were sufficiently documented to satisfy trademark standards.

Authentic Reiki

Authentic Reiki, Real Reiki, and the Radiance Technique are registered service marks of the Radiance Technique International Association, Inc. Dr. Barbara Ray, one of Hawayo Takata's twenty-two Masters, states that Mrs. Takata instructed her in the seven degrees of the Usui System of Natural Healing prior to Takata's death in 1980.

Tera Mai Reiki and Seichem

Tera Mai Reiki combines Usui Reiki and Seichem. Seichem (pronounced SAY-keem) is an Egyptian energy-based healing system. Its name was derived from the Egyptian word *sekhem*, which means "power" or "energy." Sekhem, in Seichem healing, is equivalent to ki in Reiki healing.

Together, Reiki and Seichem represent the four elements: Reiki (earth), joined with the three Seichem elements, sakara (fire), sophiel (water), and angelic light (air/ether). There are various ways of giving treatment using the four different elemental healing rays—earth, water, fire, and wind.

Tera Mai is the registered trademark of Kathleen Ann Milner (USA), author of *Reiki & Other Rays of Touch Healing*. Kathleen was originally trained in traditional Reiki and Seichem. Later, she was "led by Spirit" to use an updated attunement process and symbols, and this is how Tera Mai Reiki was created. In 1995 the Tera Mai trademark was set up to protect and maintain the integrity of these new attunements. Under the terms of the trademark, Tera Mai Masters are not permitted to perform attunements from any other Reiki or Seichem system. This assures that all attunees receive the same initiations, no matter who the teacher is. All registered Tera Mai Masters are required to adapt to any additional changes in the Tera Mai system as they are "brought in from Spirit" via Kathleen Milner.

REIKI REFLECTIONS

Many Reiki systems and names are trademarked. The owner of a trademark has the exclusive right to use it on the product or service, and any related products, that it was intended to identify.

Karuna Reiki

Karuna Reiki is the registered trademark of the International Center for Reiki Training. William Lee Rand, founder and director of the International Center for Reiki Training, worked with some of his

Reiki students to develop Karuna Reiki. Rand and his students experimented with symbols gathered from Reiki Masters with whom Rand had collaborated in his earlier travels while teaching and practicing Reiki. Karuna Reiki, also defined as Reiki of Compassion, was trademarked in 1995 by the International Center for Reiki Training. Karuna, a Sanskrit word, is used in both Hinduism and Buddhism to signify "compassionate action."

Karuna Reiki classes offer two levels, two attunements, four Master symbols, and eight treatment symbols. Rand emphasizes that he did not create the Karuna Reiki symbols. He agrees that Karuna Reiki employs some of the same symbols used by other schools and systems, but he also claims that the attunement process and intention in Karuna Reiki are different. During a Karuna Reiki treatment, the practitioner chants and intones the names of these symbols. Prior Reiki Master training is a prerequisite to taking Karuna Reiki.

Lightarian Reiki

Lightarian Reiki was introduced in 1997 through the channeling efforts of Jeannine Marie Jelm, cofounder of the Lightarian Institute for Global Human Transformation located in Tucson, Arizona. Jelm is a spiritual counselor and conscious channeler for the Ascended Masters.

Jelm claims that Lightarian Reiki is based on information revealed to her by Ascended Master Buddha. The intent of Lightarian Reiki is to awaken humanity to six higher vibrational bands of Reiki energies. Via Jelm's channeling, it has been suggested that Lightarian Reiki occupies the six highest bands of a total of eight vibrational bands within the Reiki spectrum. No symbols are used in the Lightarian Reiki system. Lightarian Reiki consists of four levels of attunements: Levels I and II, III, IV, and V and VI.

Lightarian Attunement Levels I and II

The initial Lightarian attunements for Level I and II are achieved through a guided meditation. They serve as an introduction to the energies of Ascended Master Buddha and offer the primary Lightarian Reiki principles. This guided meditation can be experienced in person, over the telephone, through e-mail, or remotely.

Lightarian Attunement Level III
The third attunement is an introduction to Gaia, the Earth Mother. Gaia's energies provide the attunee with help in his grounding and advancement of personal self-healing.

Lightarian Attunement Level IV
The fourth attunement connects the attunee to the vibrational healing energies of the God Source.

Lightarian Attunement Levels V and VI
This final attunement joins Ascended Master Sananda (called Jesus here on earth) together with Gaia, the God Source, and Ascended Master Buddha. This union of healing energies creates a visualization tool, called the Divine Healing Chamber, which can be utilized to bring about extraordinary healing results.

REIKI REFLECTIONS

Ascended Masters are enlightened spiritual beings who once lived on earth. Over the course of many lifetimes, they managed to complete all of their spiritual lessons and have ascended back to their divine source. They offer spiritual advice and compassion to those of us who are still in the physical realm by staying in spirit communication with chosen souls that are currently incarnate.

Wei Chi Tibetan Reiki

This system of Reiki is publicized as having been "rediscovered" through channeled information received by Kevin Ross Emery. The channeled entity, Wei Chi, claims that he is a 5,000-year-old Tibetan monk. Along with his brothers, Wei Chi was a creator of the original Reiki system. Wei Chi asserts that many of the original teachings have been lost through the centuries.

In this new system, the recipient and the practitioner hold dialogue before, during, and after the treatment. The practitioner not only channels Reiki's ki energies, but intuitively gleans information from the recipient as well. This information is shared with the recipient as a means to help him become a more active player, empowering the recipient to heal more deeply.

Either a third person takes notes or a tape recorder is used to record any information that is communicated during the session. There are no sequenced hand placements in Wei Chi Tibetan Reiki. The practitioner intuitively moves his hands wherever they are drawn. After the session, the practitioner and recipient discuss how it went, laying out a plan for the recipient to undertake in order to continue the healing process.

The treatment of Wei Chi Tibetan Reiki can only be performed if the recipient meets the following two conditions:

1. The recipient has to acknowledge that he is responsible for everything that happens in his life, for both good and bad, and that all life experiences teach us important lessons.
2. The recipient has to be willing to participate in his own healing.

If the recipient does not meet these requirements, the Wei Chi practitioner will refuse to treat him.

More Variations

As a result of individuals adding other healing modalities to Reiki systems already in place, the following offshoot systems have been developed as well. The inventors of these systems are really nothing more than bakers adding ingredients to spice up a cake recipe that is already sufficiently palatable. As we strive to reinvent the wheel, it is important to remember that the wheel spins effectively without any fancy bells and whistles attached to it. To fully benefit from Reiki, it is not productive to become overly absorbed in intellectual studies of the many convoluted concepts. Experiencing Reiki in its simplest form is enough.

Gendai Reiki-ho

Sensei Hiroshi Doi founded Gendai Reiki-ho. It is primarily a Japanese style of Reiki. Translated into English, Gendai Reiki-ho means "Modern Reiki Method for Healing."

However, Gendai Reiki-ho also includes influences from Western Reiki systems and other healing modalities, as well as influences from the Western Reiki systems founded by Sensei Hiroshi Doi. In his teachings, Doi explains to his students the differences in the system, clarifying which material is "traditional Japanese Reiki" and which is "Western Reiki." There are four levels of teachings in Gendai Reiki-ho: Shoden, Okuden, Shinpiden, and Gokuikaiden.

Karuna Ki

Vincent Amador developed the Karuna Ki system, also called the Way of Compassionate Energy. In no way associated with Karuna Reiki, this system is a culmination of "healing art" and "meditative practices." Amador has chosen to keep this system free of limiting trademarks, allowing teachers to add information to its basic teachings as they feel inclined.

Kundalini Reiki

Kundalini Reiki is an easy-to-use healing technique that requires no intense study or complex procedures. Its attunement process allows the chakras to be opened wider to allow kundalini energy to flow more easily and fully through your body.

Kundalini Reiki was introduced by a native of Denmark, Mr. Ole Gabrielsen, known best for his bestselling meditation CDs.

Kundalini Reiki is a direct result of Mr. Gabrielsen's communications with Ascended Master Kuthumi. Mahatma Kuthumi lived in the early nineteenth century. He was born to a Punjabi family that settled in Kashmir. Records indicate that he attended Oxford University in 1850 and is believed to have contributed "The Dream of Ravan" to *The Dublin University Magazine* around 1854. His final years were lived in seclusion in Shigatse, Tibet. Letters that he had sent to his students from Tibet are now on file with the British Museum.

REIKI REFLECTIONS

The kundalini energy, also referred to as kundalini fire, is a channel of energy that flows upward from the root chakra (located near the coccyx) to the crown chakra (located on the top of the head). Having an open kundalini indicates that there has been a complete cleansing of the chakras and that the body parts and the energy channels are unblocked.

Kundalini Reiki Level I

There are three Kundalini Reiki attunements. The first attunement opens the Reiki channel and also prepares the attunee for Level II. The crown, heart, and hand chakras are opened and strengthened.

At this stage, the attunee learns how to give a complete healing treatment and how to heal remotely.

Kundalini Reiki Level II
The second attunement is called the Kundalini Awakening. The main energy channel opens gently and the kundalini fire is lit. The flame of the kundalini reaches upward to the solar plexus chakra in preparation for the complete kundalini rising that takes place in Level III. A specific meditation is taught that increases the power of the kundalini and cleanses the chakra system.

Kundalini Reiki Level III
The third attunement is the Master Level of Kundalini Reiki. The attunee's throat, solar plexus, hara (sacral chakra), and root chakras are opened. The previous attunements are strengthened as well. A full rising of the kundalini takes place during this attunement. The student learns how to attune crystals and other objects to serve as Reiki channels, and she is taught how to pass attunements for all levels of Kundalini Reiki.

Reiki TUMMO
Another Reiki system involving the awakening of the kundalini is called Reiki TUMMO. This system is said to be very different from other Usui-based Reiki traditions and was supposedly taught by Buddha as a means to achieve enlightenment in the scope of one lifetime.

Shamballa Reiki
John Armitage developed the Shamballa Multidimensional Healing System. Shamballa is promoted as not only a system of healing, but also as a way of accelerating your spiritual development. Classes are available from Level I through Master/Teacher Level. The full system includes 352 symbols, the DNA symbol, and Mahatma initiation, and encompasses a twelve-chakra system.

A high priest at the Temple of Healing who resided in the ancient civilization of Atlantis is credited as the originator of Shamballa Reiki. This high priest, now known as Ascended Master Saint Germain, went into the far mountains away from the central temples of Atlantis, creating his own separate tribe of Atlanteans called the Inspirers. In that lifetime, Saint Germain was given twenty-two symbols.

When Atlantis was destroyed, Saint Germain journeyed with several of his people, the Inspirers, to ancient Tibet. Saint Germain and the Inspirers chose not to give the full twenty-two symbols to any individuals in that region in order to protect Reiki from possible corruption. Shamballa practitioners feel that the Reiki system, as it is practiced today, is an incomplete system. It was revealed to Dr. John Armitage by the Collective Consciousness of the Lords and Ladies of Shamballa (the Ascended Masters) that there are 352 symbols in the Shamballa Reiki System, which correspond to 352 levels, or initiations.

Rainbow Reiki

Rainbow Reiki is a spiritual way developed by Walter Lübeck as a result of his in-depth research into the many healing modalities, including Usui Reiki, shamanism, feng shui, meditation, human psychology, holistic communication sciences, and mind-body-spirit healing. The three pillars of Rainbow Reiki are love, self-responsibility, and consciousness.

Violet Flame Reiki

Violet Flame Reiki is a system of Reiki dedicated to Lady Quan Yin, the goddess of compassion and mercy. One day, while Ivy Moore was meditating upon Quan Yin and wishing to develop better healing skills using Reiki, she channeled approximately forty symbols. The focus of this Reiki system is clearing away the ego and healing with a pure heart. Usui Reiki Level II and beyond are prerequisites for learning Violet Flame Reiki.

Lady Quan Yin is one of the deities in the Buddhist tradition. She is best known as the goddess of mercy. Quan Yin's role as Buddhist Madonna is comparable to that of Mary, the mother of Jesus, in Christianity.

From a Common Source

Reiki is pure in its essence. However, the vibrational energies of Reiki, while being channeled through our bodies, blend in with our individual vibrational identities. This means that for each of us, our experiences with Reiki can be distinctly different. Different Reiki systems were ultimately derived from those varied experiences. Human nature has urged some people to challenge the past systems of Reiki and to pioneer new paths.

The roots of Reiki and the various Reiki systems that have developed since its inception are evidence that Reiki is and will continue to be an evolving energy-healing modality. The absolute essence of Reiki is constant, but it will take on different forms, depending on the personality of the practitioner who uses it.

CHAPTER 17

WHAT REIKI IS NOT

Things do not change; we change.

Henry David Thoreau

TODAY THERE ARE MORE nontraditional Reiki Masters than traditional ones. Nontraditional Reiki Master/Teachers are those who don't teach and use solely Reiki techniques but supplement their Reiki classes with teaching materials and techniques used in other healing methodologies. While there is no reason Reiki can't be used in connection with other healing practices, some students come out of these nontraditional classes confused about what truly constitutes Reiki. Often, the best way to define something is to describe in detail what that something is not. That's what this chapter covers and what you'll learn more about as you read. You'll discover the best way to use Reiki with other healing practices and how to distinguish it from other healing modalities. You'll learn more about other touch therapies that you may be interested in incorporating into your healing journey. You will also find encouragement regarding how to stay on the Reiki path.

Traditional Reiki Organizations

Considerable confusion exists as to which Usui Reiki groups or Usui Reiki systems qualify as being traditional Reiki. Depending on whom you ask, the answers will vary considerably. Arguments can be made for and against many of these groups. Here are a few that are commonly considered traditional:

- Usui Reiki Ryoho Gakkai—Usui Society in Japan
- The Reiki Alliance—Usui–Hayashi–Takata–Furumoto lineage
- The Radiance Technique International Association, Inc. (TRTIA)—Dr. Barbara Ray and Mrs. Takata started this organization in 1980
- Usui Shiki Ryoho—All Usui Reiki practitioners who trained under Takata's lineage in the West, including the Reiki Alliance members as well as other practitioners

Usui Reiki Ryoho Gakkai

Usui Reiki Ryoho Gakkai, founded by Dr. Mikao Usui, is still active today. This is primarily a secret society. It's likely that the Reiki they practice would be the closest to what Usui originally developed. However, the members do not use the term "traditional" to describe the Usui Reiki system they practice.

REIKI REFLECTIONS

The Reiki certificate that Hawayo Takata was awarded by Chujiro Hayashi certified her as a Master of Dr. Usui's Reiki System of Healing. Her certificate was signed and notarized on February 21, 1938, in Honolulu, Hawaii. This certification qualified her as an Usui Reiki Master.

The Reiki Alliance

Members of the Reiki Alliance took it upon themselves to designate Phyllis Lei Furumoto as Takata's successor, awarding her the title of Reiki Grand Master. However, Takata never officially made Furumoto or anyone else her successor.

Some Reiki Alliance members don't consider those who have attained Reiki Master Level through non–Alliance Masters to be traditional Reiki Masters. Supposedly, these Alliance members are not happy that the nonmembers never paid the $10,000 fee for mastership as required by Takata. Controversy still exists over which of these claims and allegations are true.

The Radiance Technique International Association

The Radiance Technique International Association, Inc. is a nonprofit organization run by a staff and board of directors. Dr. Ray and Mrs. Takata started this organization in 1980, although originally it was named the American Reiki Association (ARA), with Takata welcoming several hundred people in Atlanta to the ARA when it first began. In contradiction to Furumoto's claim, Dr. Barbara Ray states she was given more training along with additional information from Hawayo Takata, which no one else was made privy to. In particular, she says Takata passed on to Ray the complete teaching and activations of the seven degrees of Reiki. TRTIA trademarked the technique as Authentic Reiki, also known as Real Reiki. A review of the TRTIA website indicates that the word "traditional" does not appear. The Radiance Technique is not "traditional" in that it is taught as a science of universal energy, not based on Japanese tradition or any kind of lineage.

Reiki Is . . .	Reiki Isn't . . .
A spiritual healing art	A religion
A way of life	A one-time cure
Energy work	Massage therapy
A complementary medicine	A substitute for medical care

Traditional or Not

Some traditional Reiki Masters have become disgruntled when other Reiki Masters, who supposedly do not qualify as traditional teachers, promote themselves as traditional Reiki Masters. They feel that any Reiki Master/Teacher who has strayed from Takata's teachings in any way at all should refer to himself or herself as a nontraditional or independent teacher.

However, recent research has revealed that Hayashi modified Usui's original teachings and that Takata also taught a modified form of Reiki that strayed from what Hayashi taught, perhaps to suit her own purposes. Considering these modifications in Reiki, discussions about who should or should not call themselves traditional teachers seem pointless.

Today, a widely accepted definition of a nontraditional Reiki Master/Teacher is someone who teaches the same basic principles that Takata taught her students, but who will also include instructions for additional healing methodologies in his Reiki class. A principled Reiki instructor will inform students that any additional techniques being taught in the classroom are not Reiki. Unfortunately, some Reiki teachers don't distinguish between these additional techniques and those of Reiki as clearly as they should. In other cases, students who do not pay close enough attention to instructions during a class might come out of the class assuming that these other ideas or techniques are a part of Reiki.

Many Reiki practitioners have acquired training in a variety of healing methods. For these practitioners, Reiki is only one of several tools tucked away in their medicine bags.

For these reasons, it has become difficult today to clearly express what is distinctly Reiki and what clearly is not. Just for the record, let's review the basics of traditional Reiki classes:

- Reiki history
- Reiki principles
- Reiki attunements
- Reiki treatments
- Reiki hand placements
- Reiki symbols

What Nontraditional Classes Have to Offer

Perhaps you are inclined to seek out a nontraditional Reiki Master in order to gather additional healing tools along with the attunements and Reiki training. Because all Reiki classes are not equal, take your time researching nontraditional classes that are available. Also, if you are interested in specific healing methodologies like crystal therapy or chakra balancing, you may very well be able to find a Reiki Master who is adept in those areas as well.

On the Plus Side

Nontraditional teachers tend to have lower class fees. There are a few nontraditional teachers who even offer their services for free. If you take your time to carefully research and interview prospective nontraditional teachers, it is possible that you will find someone who has been attuned to Reiki, is very knowledgeable, and whose actions are well principled.

On the Minus Side

If you don't bother to check up on a nontraditional teacher, you could be throwing your money away when she proves to be less than knowledgeable, or worse, fraudulent. Unfortunately, there are some charlatans out there who have never been attuned to Reiki and who offer bogus attunements to others. It's important to be on your guard. Some of these corrupt teachers will even offer bogus attunements for free, simply for the thrill of deception.

REIKI REFLECTIONS

If you suspect that you have possibly received a fake attunement, don't blame yourself for being swindled. You are not the first to become a victim of a Reiki charlatan, and you will likely not be the last. Try to locate a reputable Reiki teacher in your area and begin your training over. All paths eventually lead to wisdom, including those we walk with misguided footsteps.

Distinguishing Reiki from Other Modalities

A wide variety of additional concepts are taught in nontraditional Reiki classes. These methodologies and techniques are often combined with Reiki during a treatment. As a result, the recipient will walk away from this species of Reiki treatment thinking that Reiki consists of massage, crystal therapy, and aromatherapy. But nothing could be further from the truth.

Reiki does not involve muscle manipulation, crystal therapy, psychic surgery, or chakra work. Although Reiki can be combined effectively with these and other healing methods, none of these things are Reiki.

If a recipient has come to you expecting a Reiki treatment, it is your obligation to conduct a Reiki treatment without the integration of other healing methods—unless those other methods have been mutually agreed upon. For example, if you are in the habit of combining the use of aromatherapy or flower-essence therapy when giving Reiki treatments, your recipients may assume that essential oils or essences are a part of Reiki. Act responsibly and clarify what Reiki is, and what it is not, so that there will be no lingering confusion or doubt.

Reiki and Other Healing Practices

It's important to make a distinction between Reiki and other methods of treatment, but there's no reason to separate Reiki from other healing practices. Moreover, if you are clearly relying on another healing treatment, it is not necessary to tell the recipient that Reiki is also involved. If you're giving a massage, you don't need to warn your client that you may use Reiki energies as well. For one thing, you may not actually plan to include Reiki in these types of sessions. However, Reiki has a mind of its own. It flows when and where it is needed.

Nurses and massage therapists who have been attuned to Reiki may never disclose when Reiki starts flowing from their palms as they handle their patients. Reiki will naturally kick in when it is needed and will continue to flow for as long as the recipient is subconsciously open to receiving it. Healers become accustomed to Reiki flowing freely from their hands as they perform their duties. They need not feel obligated to share this information. Hospice workers and nursing assistants who are Reiki practitioners will also notice Reiki flowing through them to the people they are assisting.

Reiki is not everything. Reiki is only one healing system, and although it would likely take more than a lifetime for a person to say he fully understands the complexities within this simple healing art, there are many other hands-on healing systems worth exploring. It is good to be open to all possibilities.

REIKI REFLECTIONS

Types of modalities that Reiki can easily be integrated with include massage therapy, reflexology, acupuncture, chiropractic care, chakra alignment, polarity therapy, and regression therapy.

Other Touch or Energy-Based Therapies

Aside from Reiki, there are many other therapies, both ancient and modern, that are based on "touch" and/or "life force." Each has its own unique history, purpose, and methodology. Techniques used in Healing Touch and Quantum-Touch healing practices are very closely related to Reiki. Hands-on healing modalities that are based on the use of ki energies, such as the Alexander Technique and shiatsu massage, involve manipulation of the body's bone structure, muscles, and skin.

Alexander Technique

The Alexander Technique is a body alignment therapy used to help recipients manage pain, relax muscular tension, learn corrective breathing techniques, and develop better postures. This technique is based on the premise that tightened muscles support misaligned bone structure, expend unnecessary energy, and create discomfort and fatigue. The Alexander Technique teacher uses his hands to gently release muscular strains and encourage correction of the bone structure so that the whole body is balanced and in good alignment.

The recipient becomes an active participant in the Alexander Technique treatment through body awareness, acquiring better posture and body movement habits—which, in turn, allow the skeletal structure to align naturally with the relaxed muscles.

Aura Clearing and Chakra Balancing

Many different techniques have been introduced in recent years that can be employed to clean "dirty" auras and correct "imbalanced" chakras. Recently, many healers have been showing increasing interest in the study of the chakras and the human energy field.

First Chakra

The first chakra, also known as the root chakra, is associated with the color red. This chakra is the grounding force that allows us to connect to the earth energies and empowers our life force. It is through this chakra that the child feels a connection with its birth mother and also the nuclear family. This area is also the place from which our survival instincts spring forth. When this chakra is misaligned, we experience confusion, distraction, and disconnection.

Second Chakra

The second chakra, also known as the sacral chakra, is associated with the colors orange and red-orange. This chakra often offers us the opportunity to acknowledge our issues regarding control, especially regarding our relationships with others. The process of creating changes in our lives through making personal choices is a function of second-chakra energy. A well-functioning second chakra helps a person maintain a healthy yin-yang (feminine-masculine) existence.

Third Chakra

The third chakra, also known as the solar plexus chakra, is associated with the color yellow. This is where our egos and intuitions reside. The healthfulness or lack of healthfulness of this chakra shapes our personal self-esteem. If you experience difficulty maintaining your personal power, it's a telltale sign that your third chakra is compromised. This intuitive chakra is also the source from which we get those "gut feelings" that signal us to take action or to avoid something. Our intuitive skills are sharpened when this chakra is functioning optimally.

Fourth Chakra

The fourth chakra, also known as the heart chakra, is associated with the colors green or pink. This chakra is considered to be the love center of our human energy system. Physical illnesses that are brought about by wounds of the heart require that an emotional healing occur along with the physical healing. Our deepest emotions, such as love, heartbreak, grief, pain, and fear, are felt strongly in this chakra. For this reason, energy-based therapies that focus on balancing the heart chakra are often the purest healing. Learning self-love is a powerful initiative to undertake in order to secure a healthy fourth chakra.

Fifth Chakra

The fifth chakra, also known as the throat chakra, is associated with the color sky blue. This chakra is our will center. It is through our speech that we express ourselves to others. The healthfulness of the fifth chakra is signified by how honestly a person expresses himself. A challenge to the throat chakra is for us to express ourselves in the most truthful manner. When we choose to speak falsehoods and half-truths, we are energetically polluting the throat chakra and violating both our bodies and spirits. Repressing our anger or displeasure by ignoring these emotions through evasive sweet talk, or keeping silent, will manifest into throat imbalances such as strep throat, laryngitis, and speech impediments.

We have all experienced that lump in our throat at times when we are unable to find the right words to speak. But when the words do begin to form, it is important that we project them clearly and truthfully with our voices. When we do not speak out, we are not only stifling our speech, but we are also stifling our heartfelt emotions. All choices we make in our lives have consequences on an energetic level, even our silences. Doing nothing and saying nothing are life choices that can affect our health.

Sixth Chakra

The sixth chakra, also known as the brow chakra, is associated with the color indigo. It is also often referred to as either the third eye or the mind center. Our mental calculations and thinking processes are functions of this chakra. We are able to evaluate our past experiences and put them into perspective through the wisdom of this chakra's actions.

Our ability to separate reality from fantasy or delusion is connected to the healthfulness of this chakra. Achieving the art of detachment outside the frame of petty-mindedness is accomplished through developing impersonal intuitive reasoning. It is through a receptive brow chakra that aura colors and other visual images are intuitively received.

Seventh Chakra

The seventh chakra, also known as the crown chakra, is associated with the color violet or white. The crown chakra is used as a mechanism for inner communication with our spiritual nature. The opening in the crown chakra serves as an entryway wherein the Universal Life Force can enter our bodies and be dispersed downward into the lower six chakras.

This chakra is often depicted as a lotus flower with its petals open to represent spiritual awakening. The crown chakra could also be considered the bottomless well from which intuitive knowledge is drawn.

Bowen Therapy

The Bowen Technique was originally developed and practiced by an Australian named Thomas Ambrose Bowen (1916–1982). Bowen Therapy is a gentle, relaxing bodywork that is administered by manipulating thumb and fingers in a rolling motion over muscles to release energy blocks. Waiting periods are incorporated between sequenced series of movements, which are conducted across specific muscles and connective tissues to alleviate different physical dis-eases. The precise, delicate movements are applied to the recipient's muscles, either directly over the skin or through light clothing. It is reported that Bowen Therapy may help to relieve the following conditions:

- Autoimmune diseases
- Digestive disorders
- Gynecological problems
- Musculoskeletal pain
- Respiratory problems

CranioSacral Therapy

CranioSacral Therapy is a type of bodywork that involves making slight adjustments to the bone and tissue of the body. This hands-on method of healing was developed by an osteopathic physician named John E. Upledger. Upledger became interested in the craniosacral system in the 1970s and began exploring previously disregarded research theorizing bone movement of the human skull. This early research was performed by Dr. William Sutherland, who is often referred to as the "father of cranial osteopathy."

CranioSacral Therapy has been compared to Reiki because of the way in which a CranioSacral Therapy session is conducted. The CranioSacral Therapy practitioner uses a gentle touch, beginning at the skull of the recipient and moving downward onto the shoulder, torso, and the lower extremities of the body. Practitioners are trained to evaluate and release any restrictions in the soft tissue surrounding the central nervous system that are creating stress or distortion.

Healing Touch

The trademarked Healing Touch Program was developed by Janet Mentgen, RN, BSN. In 1990, this program of study was accepted as a certificate program of the American Holistic Nurses Association (AHNA). The Canadian Holistic Nurses Association has endorsed it as well. In 1996, Healing Touch International, Inc. became the certifying organization for this hands-on energy-based therapy.

Healing Touch consists of six levels of training: Level I, IIA, IIB, III, IV, and V. Each level requires a commitment of several hours of instruction to gain knowledge and hands-on practice to develop Healing Touch skills. Practitioner certification can be attained after Level III. Level IV training is for the practitioner's involvement in case studies, mentoring others, and establishing client/therapist relationships, ethics, and the development of a private practice. Level V is the instructor level, intended for the certified Healing Touch practitioner to learn how to teach Healing Touch.

Huna Healing

Huna healing is more than a healing therapy; it is also a principled way of life. Huna healing is an ancient energy-work system that originated in the Hawaiian Islands. Its name is attributed to Max Freedom Long (1890–1971); *huna* is the Hawaiian word for "secret."

In its purest form, Huna healing is ancient knowledge enabling a person to connect to her highest wisdom within. Understanding and using the fundamentals, or seven principles, can help people bring about healing and harmony through the power of the mind. As an integrated healing art and earth culture, Huna is spiritual in nature. Experiencing its concepts gives us the opportunity to integrate mind, body, and spirit. One might acknowledge Huna teachings as one of nature's tools helpful in developing inner knowledge and enhancing innate psychic abilities.

Ike (ee-kay)	The world is what you think it is.
Kala	There are no limits. Everything is possible.
Makia	Energy flows where attention goes.
Manawa	Now is the moment of power.
Aloha	To love is to be happy with (someone or something).
Mana	All power comes from within.
Pono	Effectiveness is the measure of truth.

Johrei Healing

Johrei healing is a Japanese focusing and scanning technique used to dispel negativity and to increase vitality. No actual touching is involved in this healing process. The Johrei practitioner and recipient sit in chairs facing each other. The practitioner holds the palm of her hand toward the recipient while focusing and directing ki energies toward him. Energies are directed at the recipient's forehead, upper chest, and abdomen for approximately ten minutes. Then the recipient is asked to face the opposite direction, with his back to the Johrei practitioner. The practitioner focuses and directs ki energies toward the recipient's crown and the back of his head, then toward both shoulders and down the spine. Finally, the recipient returns to his original sitting position so that they are once again facing each other. The two individuals, practitioner and recipient, join together and give a silent prayer of gratitude.

The following positive effects are attributed to Johrei healing:

- It increases spiritual quality of life.
- It clears mental confusion.
- It detoxifies the physical body.
- It accelerates the process of healing.

According to the Johrei Fellowship website, "Any individual, when properly prepared, can focus this universal energy. The intensity may differ according to the level of the individual's awareness, but it is possible for any individual to focus it effectively."

Johrei healing is only one aspect of the Johrei Fellowship, which is a spiritually principled organization. Johrei was introduced to America in 1953, and Johrei Fellowship centers exist throughout the United States. The fellowship has incorporated the following Seven Spiritual Principles into its work:

1. Order
2. Gratitude
3. Purification
4. Spiritual affinity
5. Cause and effect
6. The spiritual precedes the physical
7. Oneness of the spiritual and the physical

Matrix Energetics

Matrix Energetics is a transformative system of healing combining light touch and focused intention to affect positive changes. Developed by chiropractor and naturopath Richard Barlett, DC, ND, Matrix Energetics is a technique that relies on the practitioner focusing on solutions rather than problems when treating clients. Bartlett reasons that when treating a condition, you are giving it more attention and are actually validating it, making it more "linear, predictable, and ultimately more self-aware."

A foundational assessment or tracking tool used in Matrix Energetics is the implementation of a technique called two-point. The two-point technique is used on the body of the recipient. The first point targets pain or a weakened area of the body. The second point is an energy spot detected on the body that, when touched, creates a magnetic pull from the first point. The practitioner keeps one hand firmly in place on the first point while his other hand seeks out a polarizing second point. Once found, the Matrix Energetics practitioner drags his fingers across the recipient's skin from the second point to the first point while mentally linking the two points together.

Polarity Therapy

Randolph Stone, DO, DC, ND (1890–1981), developed Polarity Therapy. In 1984, a national organization, the American Polarity Therapy Association, was established to practice and teach this healing system. Polarity Therapy involves energy-based bodywork, nutrition, exercise, and self-awareness. The Polarity Therapy practitioner assesses the recipient's energetic attributes using touch, observation, and interview methods. Application of touching can range from light touch to medium or firm pressure. The techniques used in this therapy are complementary to many other holistic health systems.

Pranic Healing

Pranic Healing is a nontouch energy-based technique that accelerates the healing process through the use of "life force" being directed to the part of the physical body that needs healing. In order to locate blockages of ki, the Pranic Healing practitioner scans the recipient's aura or "energy field." Ki energies are then projected through the Pranic Healing practitioner's palm chakras to cleanse, energize, and revitalize the problematic area.

Grand Master Choa Kok Sui founded Pranic Healing as a result of spending more than eighteen years researching and studying esoteric sciences. He has written several books about his findings, including *Miracles Through Pranic Healing* and *Advanced Pranic Healing*.

Stephen Co is a senior disciple of Grand Master Choa Kok Sui and the world's foremost authority in Pranic Healing. In his Pranic Healing workshops, Co teaches a simple exercise that activates the palm chakras.

VortexHealing

VortexHealing is a spiritually oriented healing system that is based on the premise that all of our ailments are the result of us experiencing separation from the divine consciousness. In 1995, Ric Weinman, founder of VortexHealing, began teaching this healing art in order to assist the process of spiritual awakening.

Shiatsu Massage

Shiatsu, also known as acupressure, is a finger-pressure massage technique that is sometimes confused with acupuncture. Although both shiatsu massage therapy and acupuncture are founded on the Chinese meridian system, there are no needle pokes involved with shiatsu. Massage techniques like tapping, squeezing, rubbing, and applied pressure are applied along the meridians to reintroduce the optimal flow of ki.

Energy Pathways

Meridians are the pathways of ki and blood flow through the body. When a person's overall health is good, ki will flow continuously from one meridian to another. Any break in the flow is an indication of imbalance. Whenever a person's vitality or energy is recognizably diminished, this signifies that the body's organs or tissues are functioning poorly, and therefore, the ki flow is insufficient.

The Meridian Healing System

The meridian healing system is based on the concept that an insufficient supply of ki compromises a person's immune system, making her vulnerable to dis-ease. Restoring the ki is the ultimate goal in restoring overall health and well-being to the individual. Acupuncturists, Chinese herbalists, and shiatsu massage therapists assist clients in repairing dysfunctional areas within the meridian system in order to restore a natural balance.

Twelve Major Meridians

There are twelve major meridians that correspond to specific human organs: kidneys, liver, spleen, heart, lungs, pericardium, bladder, gallbladder, stomach, small and large intestines, and the triple burner (body temperature regulator). Yin meridians flow upward. Yang meridians flow downward. Pathways corresponding to the yang organ are often used to treat disorders of its related yin organ.

CORRESPONDING YIN AND YANG ORGANS

Yin Organs	Yang Organs
Lungs	Large intestine
Pericardium	Triple burner
Heart	Small intestine
Spleen	Stomach
Liver	Gallbladder
Kidney	Bladder

Therapeutic Touch

Therapeutic Touch is considered a modern version of an array of ancient energy-based healing methods. Dolores Krieger, PhD, RN, and Dora van Gelder Kunz developed this healing system. Therapeutic Touch was originally taught to a group of graduate nurses in 1972 and today is still primarily practiced among healthcare professionals. However, the training is not exclusive to nurses and doctors—it is also available to anyone else who wishes to learn it.

A basic Therapeutic Touch workshop consists of approximately twelve classroom hours. To qualify as a Therapeutic Touch practitioner, a student must take the intermediate-level workshop and be mentored for twelve months under the care of a qualified Therapeutic Touch practitioner/teacher.

The Therapeutic Touch practitioner applies gentle sweeping movements with his hands a few inches over the recipient's body to clear away imbalances and revitalize the recipient's personal energy. Its primary purposes are to manage pain and promote healing.

The Trager Approach
The Trager Approach is a tension-reducing treatment involving gentle rocking and vibrating movements. The intention of a Trager treatment is to release built-up patterns of tension in the joints and muscles of the body, creating a sense of deep relaxation within the recipient. The recipient remains passive throughout the process and is encouraged to relax and "let go" physically, mentally, and emotionally. Following treatment, simple exercises called Mentastics are given to the recipient for home use. These exercises are meant to reinforce the subconscious messages initiated during treatment.

The Trager Approach has been reported to ease or manage a wide range of conditions, including stress, back and neck pain, limited movement, muscle spasms, depression, headaches, multiple sclerosis, post-polio syndrome, cerebral palsy, sports-related injuries, Parkinson's disease, carpal tunnel syndrome, and fibromyalgia.

Milton Trager, MD (1908–1997), who developed the Trager Approach, became interested in the structure and function of the body as a result of the childhood congenital spinal deformity that he overcame. In 1980, Trager established the Trager Institute with the help of Betty Fuller.

Quantum-Touch
Quantum-Touch is a vibrational touch therapy that incorporates touch, breath work, and body-awareness meditations. Its concepts are closely related to Polarity Therapy. It is primarily a light-touch energy therapy, but it is secondarily promoted as a therapy that

helps bones to spontaneously adjust to their proper alignment. Richard Gordon developed Quantum-Touch therapy and published a book on this therapy, *Quantum-Touch: The Power to Heal.*

The Quantum-Touch healing process involves the practitioner "running energy" into the recipient's body. Often, practitioners employ a technique that is known as "sandwiching" or "the hand sandwich." Sandwiching means that the practitioner will use her hands to sandwich the part of the recipient's body that is to be treated. One hand will be placed on one side of the body part and the other hand will be placed on the other side. Another technique that is used for "running energy" into very small areas is to create a tripod using the thumb, forefinger, and middle finger. This is meant to help get the practitioner's hands closer to the source of pain. Advanced techniques used in this system include harmonic toning, spinning the chakras, structural alignment, and distance healing.

Staying on the Reiki Path

While it is tempting to explore all the possible healing modalities, it takes time, effort, and energy just to understand one! So while it is fine to be open to other ideas and information, and to use practices you already know, remember that you'll get more out of Reiki the more you put into it.

Reiki history is steeped in tradition. Some Reiki practitioners are questioning parts of the tradition that have been proved less than accurate. As a result, new ways of practicing Reiki are constantly evolving. Today, Reiki continues to thrive in the healing community because its healing aspects stand by themselves. Choosing to take a nontraditional path in the study of Reiki does have its merits. However, we need to be cautious, since it is likely that there will always be individuals who will misrepresent Reiki for their own self-interests.

FREQUENTLY ASKED QUESTIONS

What is Reiki?

Reiki is a natural healing system designed to assist in healing and help achieve balance. Reiki is administered by a practitioner, who serves as a conduit through which the Universal Life Energy can be transmitted to the recipient, by either hands-on or distance healing techniques. Practitioners may also practice Reiki self-treatments.

How does Reiki energy flow?

Reiki flows through our palms at different rates of speed, depending on various factors such as the extent of the recipient's illness, degree of blockage, and his or her readiness to accept change.

How can I best understand Reiki?

The best way to understand and appreciate Reiki is to experience it by having a full-body Reiki treatment. Reiki is for everyone, and it is available to anyone who wants it.

Is Reiki a form of faith healing?

No, Reiki is not a religion, nor is it based on the acceptance of any religious doctrine. Having a belief system is not a requirement for Reiki to work. Reiki does not infringe on anyone's right to believe what he or she wishes. However, Reiki's principles are spiritual in nature and do encourage spiritual empowerment and growth.

Can Reiki be learned from a book?

Becoming a Reiki practitioner is not something you can do on your own through reading a how-to book or watching an instructional video. Receiving Reiki attunements and training can be achieved in a one-day or two-day workshop. Access to Reiki is easy. All you have to do is seek out a Reiki Master in your area who is willing to work with you.

Is Reiki for everyone?

Reiki is for everyone, but not everyone is for Reiki. Some people are simply not as open to Reiki as others.

Who can benefit from a Reiki treatment?

Reiki's gift of increased energy and vitality can be extended to anyone. It doesn't matter what a person's gender, race, intelligence, or financial status is. Reiki is not a healing energy reserved only for the elite, wealthy, educated, or spiritually evolved.

What does Reiki feel like?

Common Reiki sensations are heat or coolness, "pins and needles," vibrational buzzing, electrical sparks, numbness, throbbing, itchiness, and drowsiness.

What is a Reiki attunement?

A Reiki attunement is a ritual performed by a Reiki Master. The ritual involves energetic placement of Reiki symbols, through a specific set of sequenced actions, into the student's crown and palms.

What types of changes can I expect following my Reiki attunement?

Changes will vary from person to person, so it's impossible to predict how any one individual will react to being attuned. Changes begin to take place as soon as Reiki is introduced into the body and begins its balancing process. Reiki works to bring about only positive changes, but these changes may offer challenges while the transformation is occurring.

Will I know when Reiki is working?

Some people know when Reiki is working because they notice shifts of energies occurring. However, some people don't feel anything when giving or receiving Reiki. Just because you don't feel anything, don't assume that nothing is happening. Trust that Reiki is working.

What if my hands don't feel hot?

Experiencing hot hands is a common experience reported by Reiki practitioners. However, each person's experience with Reiki is unique. You may not experience hot hands, so don't look for it as verification that Reiki is flowing through them.

I feel balls of energy collecting in my hands. What is that all about?

When excess Reiki energies build up in your palms, it may be an indication that a Reiki self-treatment is needed. Take advantage of this excess of energy in your hands and place your hands on your body. Allowing the Reiki to flow into your body should help reduce or release the ball of energy from your palms.

Will Reiki ever run out?

When you are giving a Reiki treatment to someone, you are giving of your time and your intent to assist, but you are not giving away any of your own energy. Reiki is in infinite supply. It never runs out.

Does nutrition play a role in Reiki?

Definitely! Having optimal health is essential for practicing Reiki, and eating nutritional meals regularly is essential for optimal health. Eating five or six small-portion meals each day is recommended over eating just two or three large meals.

What is the purpose of the Reiki hand placements?

Emphasis is placed on devoting five minutes on each hand placement so that no part of the body is neglected and to ensure that each body part is given equal consideration. After practicing these twelve hand placements in the traditional sequences for a period of time, you will likely deviate from them to some degree and begin to acquire your own methodology in placing your hands on the body while listening to your inner dialogue.

How often should I conduct self-treatments?
Newly attuned Reiki Level I practitioners will benefit from doing full-body sessions daily for the first four to six weeks. After those first weeks, following a regimen of one or two full-body self-treatments each week is prudent.

Are there any limitations to Reiki?
The only limitations that can block Reiki are those we create, consciously or subconsciously, through a lack of trust or belief in the potential of Reiki treatments to improve our balance or conditions of health.

Do I need to direct the flow of Reiki?
Reiki will automatically go to wherever it needs to go with no mental involvement of either the practitioner or the recipient. However, when mental intention is used, a linear pathway is opened. This cleared route allows Reiki to flow more effectively to that part of the body where attention is most desired.

Now that I'm a Reiki practitioner, am I obligated to treat others?
You are under no obligation to treat others every time it is requested of you. You have the right to refuse treatment to anyone, without justifying your feelings. Anytime you feel strongly that you do not want to give a Reiki treatment to someone, accept those feelings without hesitation and politely refuse.

What purpose do Reiki symbols serve?
Independently, each Reiki symbol has its own unique purposes. The combined function of these symbols is to provide Reiki practitioners with focal points for their healing intentions.

Why is Reiki called "smart energy"?
Reiki is an intelligent energy because it knows which areas of the body most need healing and will automatically flow to specific areas where suffering or imbalance is prevalent.

What is a Reiki share?
A Reiki share is a time when Reiki practitioners gather together to socialize and to participate in group healing treatments. The main purpose of the share is to give and receive Reiki in a casual atmosphere of friendship, honor, and devotion.

Why did I start crying during my Reiki treatment?
Occasionally a person will experience an intense emotional release during or after a Reiki treatment. These types of emotional releases may be expressed through crying, screaming, coughing, laughing, or other reactions. Emotional releases help carry the person through the hurts and discomforts associated with the feelings that arise during a Reiki session.

Why is it important to sweep the recipient's auric field after a Reiki treatment?
Sweeping or combing through the recipient's auric field clears it of any energetic debris that has lifted from the physical body during the treatment. It is also recommended that you clear your healing space between Reiki treatments so that you don't have any negative or stagnant energies lingering in any part of the room.

Is it safe to treat children with Reiki?
Reiki's gentle and noninvasive nature is perfect for treating the ills and upsets of young children. Children are extremely receptive to Reiki's positive effects and will normally welcome it without any apprehension.

How important is it to attain the Master Level of training?
Being certified in the highest level does not necessarily reflect superior knowledge. It is through the continued practice of Reiki that one becomes proficient. The Level I practitioner who uses Reiki daily will be more aware of how Reiki works than a Level III or Master Level Reiki practitioner who seldom conducts treatments.

GLOSSARY OF TERMS

absentia treatment:
A specially formulated Reiki treatment applied whenever treating an individual or group of individuals who are not physically present. A variety of items can be used as focal points while sending an absentia treatment: healing lists, photographs, teddy bear surrogates, and so forth. Absentia treatment is also known as distance healing or long-distance healing.

Advanced Reiki Training (ART):
This is the third level of training, also called Level IIIa, of the Usui/Tibetan Reiki System. ART consists of a variety of add-on techniques such as the use of crystal grids, spirit guides, healing attunements, psychic surgeries, meditations, and Tibetan symbols.

Akashic Records:
People who believe in reincarnation believe that all lifetimes—past, present, and future—are "recorded" and are constantly being updated. These recordings are stored in the Akashic Records, which are said to exist in an etheric dimension beyond the earth's atmosphere. It is said that everything that has ever happened since the beginning of time (every event, every thought, every action, every feeling) is recorded there. The term *akasha* is derived from the Sanskrit word for "ether." Akashic Records are also known as Akasha Chronicles or Akashic Library.

attunement:
Attunement is the empowerment ritual used to awaken the Reiki energies that lie dormant in everyone's body at birth. Reiki symbols are placed into the attunee's crown and palms. It is through the attunement process that Reiki is passed from teacher to student. Attunement may also be referred to as empowerment or initiation.

booster attunements:
Booster attunements are Reiki attunements that are given to a Reiki practitioner as a "turbocharge" to

help get the Reiki flowing whenever it is dormant or blocked. The Reiki Master can use the Hui Yin attunement as a booster attunement for any level practitioner.

Byosen Reikan Ho:
Byosen Reikan Ho is a scanning technique that is used to detect dis-eases and imbalances, including those that have not yet manifested in the body. It is also used to treat residual toxins from past illnesses and as a preventative measure against the reoccurrence of past illnesses.

chakras:
Also known as energy vortexes, or wheels of light, chakras are funnel-shaped centers within our bodies that serve as intake and outflow mechanisms to control the flow of ki energies that sustain us. Open and functioning chakras spin clockwise, allowing energy to vitalize our auras and nourish our physical bodies. There are seven major chakras and twenty-one minor chakras.

Cho Ku Rei:
This is the first symbol used in Reiki. It is generally called the Power symbol. In hands-on treatments, the Cho Ku Rei is often applied by tracing it in the air counterclockwise in order to increase power. Some practitioners also draw or visualize it in a clockwise motion, to decrease the flow of energy. The Cho Ku Rei symbol can be applied to help get the Reiki "juices" flowing when the energy flow has slowed down or become blocked. When it is used for absentia healings, it is drawn or visualized to act as the "light switch" that turns the Reiki on.

Dai Ko Myo:
This is the Reiki symbol that represents the Usui Master symbol; it is also known as a Soul Healer. It is revealed to the Reiki student at the third-degree level.

Gakkai:
The Usui Reiki Ryoho Gakkai was the original Reiki organization that Dr. Mikao Usui founded in Japan. It is still active today. In Japanese, *gakkai* means "society."

Hon Sha Ze Sho Nen:
The Hon Sha Ze Sho Nen is the third symbol used in Reiki. It is also known as the Pagoda symbol and the Connection symbol. Primary functions of this symbol are sending absentia treatments, inner-child work, healing addictions, and reviewing Akashic Records.

Hui Yin Position:
The Reiki Master holds this position when passing attunements. The vaginal muscles (of female masters) and anus are contracted, blocking air from entering the vagina and rectum. While holding the Hui Yin, the tongue is pressed against the roof of the mouth, with the tip of the tongue slightly touching the gap between the back of the two front teeth. A deep breath is taken and held for two to four minutes.

human energy field (HEF):
The human energy field is more commonly known as the aura. It is the energy body, or bubble of energy, that surrounds the physical body. It consists of seven layers, and each layer carries its own unique level of frequency.

kanji:
Modified Chinese characters used in the Japanese writing system; Reiki symbols are derived from kanji. Kanji characters are pictograms that represent entire ideas or words, rather than merely alphabetic letters or syllables of words.

ki:
The life force or living energy that connects us to all there is and sustains our life breath. While the Chinese refer to the life force as chi, or qi, in Japan this living energy is called ki. The Hindus know it as prana, the Greeks as pneuma, the Polynesians as mana, and the Egyptians as ka.

kundalini:
Literally "coiled," like a bedspring, the kundalini is considered to be the creative energy housed at the base of the spine. As the kundalini is awakened and moves upward through the chakra system, a person's consciousness changes. Kundalini is also referred to as the Fire Serpent.

Okuden:
In the traditional Japanese system of Reiki, Okuden is the equivalent to Usui Reiki Level II in the Western teachings.

practitioner:
All levels of Reiki attunees are referred to as Reiki practitioners, meaning that they practice Reiki. You can also refer to Reiki practitioners as healers or Reiki facilitators.

Radiance Technique:
This system is based on secret information that Dr. Barbara Ray, one of Takata's twenty-two initiates, says was entrusted to her by Takata prior to Takata's death in 1980. The Radiance Technique is also trademarked as Real Reiki and Authentic Reiki.

Raku:
This Reiki symbol is used to finalize the attunement process. Its purpose is to lock the newly added energies within the Reiki initiate. The Raku is also known as the Lightning Bolt and the Completion symbol.

Reiji Ho:
This is the intuitive ability to locate imbalances in the body without touching it. The person's hands are intuitively led to areas and specific spots on which to lay their hands in order to facilitate a healing. This is the technique that was taught in Japan to Reiki students before the hand placements were developed.

Reiju:
Reiju is the original empowerment or initiation process used by Dr. Mikao Usui to pass Reiki energy on to his students. Reiju eventually developed into the Reiki attunement process that is recognized in the West.

The Reiki Alliance:
The Reiki Alliance is an international community of Reiki Masters of Usui Shiki Ryoho that was formed in 1983. The Reiki Alliance acknowledges the lineage of Mikao Usui, Chujiro Hayashi, Hawayo Takata, and Phyllis Lei Furumoto.

Reiki Principles:
The Reiki principles are a series of five principles, creeds, or precepts written by the Meiji Emperor that were adopted by Usui in Reiki Ryoho. There are many different variations of these five basic principles used by Reiki practitioners today.

Sei Hei Ki:
Sei Hei Ki is the second Reiki symbol. It is also known as the Dragon and the Harmony symbol. Its purposes include emotional healings, purification, clearing, and protection.

sensei:
A Japanese word for "teacher."

Shinpiden:
In the traditional Japanese system of Reiki, Shinpiden is the equivalent to Usui Reiki Master/Teacher Level in the Western teachings.

Shoden:
In the traditional Japanese system of Reiki, Shoden is the equivalent to Usui Reiki Level I in the Western teachings.

Usui Shiki Ryoho:
The Japanese system of natural healing that originated from the Reiki System of Healing, as developed by Dr. Mikao Usui. It was adopted and further adapted by Chujiro Hayashi and Hawayo Takata. Usui Shiki Ryoho has since evolved into many different Reiki healing systems that draw from the same energy source.

ADDITIONAL RESOURCES

Further Readings

Books

A-Z of Reiki Pocketbook, by Bronwen Stiene and Frans Stiene (UK: O Books, John Hunt Publishing, 2006).

All Love: A Guidebook for Healing With Sekhem-Seichim-Reiki and SKHM, by Diane Ruth Shewmaker (WA: Celestial Wellspring Publications, 1999).

Anatomy of the Spirit: The Seven Stages of Power and Healing, by Caroline Myss, PhD (NY: Three Rivers Press, 1996).

The Creative Journal: The Art of Finding Yourself, by Lucia Capacchione, PhD, ATR (OH: Swallow Press/Ohio University Press, 1979).

Energy Medicine: Balancing Your Body's Energies for Optimal Health, Joy and Vitality, by Donna Eden and David Feinstein, PhD (NY: Tarcher, 2008).

Essential Reiki: A Complete Guide to an Ancient Healing Art, by Diane Stein (CA: Crossing Press, 1995).

The Everything® Reiki Book, by Phylameana lila Désy (MA: Adams Media, 2004).

Flower Essence Repertory, by Patricia Kaminski and Richard Katz (CA: The Flower Essence Society, Revised Edition, 1994).

Hands of Light: A Guide to Healing Through the Human Energy Field, by Barbara Ann Brennan (NY: Bantam Books, 1988).

The Illustrated Encyclopedia of Healing Remedies, by C. Norman Shealy, MD, PhD (Dorset, England: Element Books Limited, 1998).

Love Is in the Earth: A Kaleidoscope of Crystals, by Melody (CO: Earth-Love Publishing House, 1995).

Matrix Energetics: The Science and Art of Transformation, by Richard Bartlett, DC, ND (NY: Atria Books, 2007).

The Meditation Sourcebook: Meditation for Mortals, by Holly Sumner, PhD (IL: Lowell House, 1999).

The Power of Reiki: An Ancient Hands-on Healing Technique, by Tanmaya Honervogt (NY: Henry Holt, 1998).

Quantum-Touch: The Power to Heal, Revised Edition, by Richard Gordon (CA: North Atlantic Books, 2002).

Reiki and the Healing Buddha, by Maureen J. Kelly (WI: Lotus Press, 2000).

Reiki Nurse: My Life As a Nurse, and How Reiki Changed It, by Meredith Kendall, RN, MSN (e-book: Booklocker.com, 2009).

Reiki Shamanism: A Guide to Out-of-Body Healing, by Jim PathFinder Ewing (Findhorn, Scotland: Findhorn Press, 2008).

Reiki: A Way of Life, by Patricia Rose Upczak (CO: Synchronicity Publishing, 1999).

Reiki: Hawayo Takata's Story, by Helen J. Haberly (MD: Archedigm Publications, 1990).

Reiki: The Legacy of Dr. Usui, by Frank Arjava Petter (WI: Lotus Press, 1998).

Soul-Level Healing: Techniques to Peel Away the Layers, by Jillian Smith, CHt, CMH (IA: Thinkers' Press, 1996).

The Spirit of Reiki: The Complete Handbook of the Reiki System, by Walter Lübeck, Frank Arjava Petter, and William Lee Rand (WI: Lotus Press, 2001).

Tails of a Healer: Animals, Reiki & Shamanism, by Rose De Dan (IN: AuthorHouse, 2007).

Vibrational Medicine: The #1 Handbook of Subtle-Energy Therapies, Third Edition, by Richard Gerber, MD (VT: Bear & Company, 2001).

Wheels of Light: Chakras, Auras, and the Healing Energy of the Body, by Rosalyn L. Bruyere (NY: Fireside, 1994).

Online Connections

Reiki Associations

Australian Reiki Connection (ARC)
www.australianreikiconnection.com.au

Canadian Reiki Association
www.reiki.ca

Christ the Healer UCC (United Church of Christ)
http://cthgathering.org/reiki

International Association of Reiki Professionals (IARP)
www.iarpreiki.org

The International Center for Reiki Training
www.reiki.org

The John Harvey Gray Center for Reiki Healing
www.learnreiki.org

The Radiance Technique International Association, Inc. (TRTIA)
www.trtia.org

The Reiki Alliance
www.reikialliance.com

The Reiki Association
www.reikiassociation.org.uk

The Reiki Council
www.reikicouncil.org.uk

Reiki for Christians
www.christianreiki.org

Reiki Healing Connection
www.reikienergy.com

The UK Reiki Federation
www.reikifed.co.uk

Online Periodicals

Reiki News Magazine
www.reikiwebstore.com/
SearchResult.cfm?CategoryID=10

The Reiki Times
*www.iarpreiki.org/The_ Reiki_*
Times_ Magazine

Touch: The Reiki Association
Community Magazine
www.reikiassociation.org.uk

Reiki Masters

Adonea (formerly Light and Adonea)
www.angelfire.com/az/SpiritMatters

Rick Bockner
www.harbydarmusic.com/about-rick

Fran Brown, now deceased
www.reikifranbrown.com

Robert Fueston
www.robertfueston.com

Phyllis Lei Furumoto
www.usuishikiryohoreiki.com /ogm/
phyllis-paul/

Lourdes Gray
http://learnreiki.org/lourdes-gray
.htm

David Herron / The Reiki Page
http://reiki.7gen.com/

Walter Lübeck
www.rainbowreikiusa.com/
Walter-Luebeck.html

Serena Lumiere
http://seedreiki.reiki.com/serena

Paul and Susan Mitchell
http://reikihealingarts.com/about-us

Frank Arjava Petter
www.reikidharma.com

William Lee Rand
www.reiki.org/ReikiClasses/
teachers/rand.html

Barbara Ray, PhD
www.trtia.org/histpers.html

Diane Stein
www.dianestein.net

Reiki Systems

Authentic Reiki
www.authenticreiki.org

Karuna Reiki
www.reiki.org/karunareiki/
karunahomepage.html

The International Center for Reiki
Training
www.reiki.org/karunareiki/
karunahomepage.html

Kundalini Reiki
Kundalini Mastery
www.kundalinireiki.com

Lightarian Reiki
Lightarian Institute
www.lightarian.com

Rainbow Reiki
Reiki Do Institute International
www.rainbowreikiusa.com

Reiki TUMMO
www.padmacahaya.com

Seichem
The Reiki and Seichem Association
www.reikiseichem.org

Tera Mai Reiki Healing
www.reikihealing.com.au

Violet Flame Reiki
www.powerattunements.com/violet

Other Healing Modalities

Alexander Technique
www.alexandertechnique.com.au

Bowen Therapy
Gerri Shapiro
www.miraclepainrelief.com

Healing Touch Program
Healing Touch International, Inc.
www.healingtouch.net

Huna Healing
www.huna.org

Polarity Therapy (American Polarity
Therapy Association)
www.polaritytherapy.org

Pranic Healing
www.pranichealing.com

Quantum-Touch
www.quantumtouch.com

Therapeutic Touch
www.therapeutic-touch.org

Trager Approach (United States
Trager Association)
www.tragerus.org

VortexHealing
www.vortexhealing.com

Reiki Blogs

Everything Reiki
http://everythingreiki.com

The Reiki Digest
http://reikidigest.blogspot.com

Reiki, Medicine & Self Care
www.ReikiInMedicine.org/reiki-blog

Reiki Nurse
http://meredithkendall.blogspot.com

Reikified!
http://reikified.com

We Are One World Healing
http://therapeuticreiki.com/blog

Reiki Facebook Pages

Everything Reiki
www.facebook.com/everything.reiki

Reiki Talk Show with Phyllis Lei
Furumoto
www.facebook.com/ReikiTalkShow
.PhyllisLeiFurumoto

Reiki, Medicine and Self-Care
www.facebook.com/ReikiMed

Reiki: Pure and Simple
www.facebook.com/reiki
.pureandsimple

Reiki Practitioners on Twitter

Rose De Dan
www.twitter.com/WildReikiShaman

Phylameana lila Désy
www.twitter.com/phylameana

Pamir Kiciman
www.twitter.com/gassho

Rhonda Kuykendall-Ja
www.twitter.com/rhondakj

Alice Langholt
www.twitter.com/reikiawakening

Astrid Lee
www.twitter.com/ReikiTeacher

Pamela Miles
www.twitter.com/wellth

Reiki Chats and Chatrooms

The God Light Reiki Chat
www.thegodlight.co.uk/god6.htm

The Halls of Reiki Chat Room
http://pub18.bravenet.com/chat/
show.php/1544305713

Reiki Communities

Regional Reiki Shares
http://healing.about.com/od/
reiki/a/reiki-circles-by-region.htm

The Reiki Learning Lounge
www.reikilearninglounge.com/forum

Yahoo Reiki Groups
https://groups.yahoo.com/neo/
search?query=reiki

Reiki Research

The Center for Reiki Research
www.centerforreikiresearch.com

National Center for Complementary
and Integrative Health
http://nccam.nih.gov/health/
whatiscam

ScienceDaily
www.sciencedaily.com

Childbirth Resources

Sacred Childbirth with Reiki
www.sacredchildbirthwithreiki.org

Animals and Reiki

Reiki Fur Babies
www.reikifurbabies.com

Wild Reiki and Shamanic Healing
www.reikishamanic.com

Other Related Web Resources

Alexandria Healing Centre
www.alexandriahealing.co.uk

The Dr. Oz Show
www.doctoroz.com

Highly Sensitive People
http://highlysensitivepeople.com

Japanese Kanji
www.thejapanesepage.com

The Upledger Institute
www.upledger.com

Usui Reiki Ryoho Gakkai
www.aetw.org/reiki_gakkai.html

INDEX

A

Absentia treatments, 90–102, 121, 183
Acceptance, 11–12
Acupressure, 217–18
Advanced Reiki Training (ART), 189–90
Akashic Records, 93, 184
Alexander Technique, 207, 208
Alone time, 35–36
Amador, Vincent, 195
American Reiki Association (ARA), 202
Angelic beings, 24, 127–29
Anxiety, 88, 121–22, 141
Armitage, John, 197, 198
Aromatherapy, 206
Ascended Masters, 24, 193, 198
Astral connections, 99
Atlantis, 198
Attire, 40–41
Attunement process, 28–37, 127, 137, 153, 162–63, 222
Attunements
    benefits of, 36–37
    for children, 158–59
    highs and lows of, 35
    Hui Yin, 34
    number of, 34
    passage of, from Master to student, 14
    purification period after, 34–36
Aura
    clearing, 83, 208–11
    smudging, 40
Aura bath, 39–40
Auric field, clearing, 135–36, 225
Authentic Reiki, 190

B

Back rub massage, 154–55
Baking soda, 39
Balance, 88
Bartlett, Richard, 215
Bathing, 39–40
Blanket, 43
Bleeding injuries, 119
Blockages, 24
Body
    cleansing your, 39–40
    emotional, 117
    emotional centers of the, 130–32
    imbalances in, 139
    mental, 117
    natural healing ability of, 89
    nourishing your, 41–42
    PEMS, 116–17
    physical, 117
    spiritual, 117
Bolster, 43
Book of Life, 93
Boundaries, creating, 84
Bowen, Thomas Ambrose, 212
Bowen Technique, 212
Breath awareness exercises, 142–43
Broken bones, 118
Brow chakra, 211
Bruises, 118
Buddha, 197
Bumps, 118
Burnout, 87
Burns, 118–19
Byosen Reikan Ho, 26

G

H

I

J

K

L

M

N

O

P

Q

R